1987 Nursing Photobook Annual

NURSING87 BOOKS™
SPRINGHOUSE CORPORATION
SPRINGHOUSE, PENNSYLVANIA

Nursing87 Books™

NURSING PHOTOBOOK™ SERIES
Providing Respiratory Care
Managing I.V. Therapy
Dealing with Emergencies
Giving Medications
Assessing Your Patients
Using Monitors
Providing Early Mobility
Giving Cardiac Care
Performing GI Procedures
Implementing Urologic Procedures
Controlling Infection
Ensuring Intensive Care
Coping with Neurologic Disorders
Caring for Surgical Patients
Working with Orthopedic Patients
Nursing Pediatric Patients
Helping Geriatric Patients
Attending Ob/Gyn Patients
Aiding Ambulatory Patients
Carrying Out Special Procedures

NURSE REVIEW™ SERIES
Cardiac Problems
Respiratory Problems
Gastrointestinal Problems
Neurologic Problems
Vascular Problems
Genitourinary Problems
Endocrine Problems
Musculoskeletal Problems

NURSING NOW™ SERIES
Shock   Cardiac Crises
Hypertension   Respiratory Emergencies
Drug Interactions   Pain

NEW NURSING SKILLBOOK™ SERIES
Giving Emergency Care Competently
Monitoring Fluid and Electrolytes Precisely
Assessing Vital Functions Accurately
Coping with Neurologic Problems Proficiently
Reading EKGs Correctly
Combatting Cardiovascular Diseases Skillfully
Nursing Critically Ill Patients Confidently
Dealing with Death and Dying
Managing Diabetes Properly
Giving Cardiovascular Drugs Safely

NURSE'S REFERENCE LIBRARY®
Diseases   Definitions
Diagnostics   Practices
Drugs   Emergencies
Assessment   Signs & Symptoms
Procedures   Patient Teaching

NURSE'S CLINICAL LIBRARY®
Cardiovascular Disorders
Respiratory Disorders
Endocrine Disorders
Neurologic Disorders
Renal and Urologic Disorders
Gastrointestinal Disorders
Neoplastic Disorders
Immune Disorders

CLINICAL POCKET MANUAL™ SERIES
Diagnostic Tests   Critical Care
Emergency Care   Neurologic Care
Fluids and Electrolytes Surgical Care
Signs and Symptoms   Medications and I.V.s
Cardiovascular Care   Ob/Gyn Care
Respiratory Care   Pediatric Care

Nursing87 DRUG HANDBOOK™

Nursing Yearbook87

**Springhouse Corporation
Book Division**

CHAIRMAN
Eugene W. Jackson

VICE-CHAIRMAN
Daniel L. Cheney

PRESIDENT
Warren R. Erhardt

VICE-PRESIDENT AND DIRECTOR
William L. Gibson

VICE-PRESIDENT,
BOOK OPERATIONS
Thomas A. Temple

VICE-PRESIDENT, PRODUCTION
AND PURCHASING
Bacil Guiley

PROGRAM DIRECTOR
Jean Robinson

ART DIRECTOR
John Hubbard

Staff for this Volume

BOOK EDITOR
Katherine W. Carey

CLINICAL EDITOR
Diane Schweisguth, RN, BSN, CCRN, CEN

EDITOR
Kathy Goldberg

PHOTOGRAPHER
Paul A. Cohen

PROJECT COORDINATOR
Aline S. Miller

SENIOR DESIGNER
Jacalyn Bove Facciolo

EDITORIAL SERVICES MANAGER
David R. Moreau

COPY EDITORS
Diane M. Labus
Doris Weinstock
Debra Young

DRUG INFORMATION MANAGER
Larry Neil Gever, RPh, PharmD

PRODUCTION COORDINATOR
Maureen B. Carmichael

ACQUISITIONS
Margaret L. Belcher, RN, BSN

ADMINISTRATIVE ASSISTANT
Betty Anne McBeath

CONTRIBUTING DESIGNER
Julie Carleton Barlow

ART PRODUCTION MANAGER
Robert Perry

ARTISTS
Donald G. Knauss
Mark Marcin
Bob Wieder

ILLUSTRATORS
Dan Fione
Robert Jackson

TYPOGRAPHY MANAGER
David C. Kosten

TYPOGRAPHY ASSISTANTS
Elizabeth A. DiCicco
Diane Paluba
Nancy Wirs

SENIOR PRODUCTION MANAGER
Deborah C. Meiris

ASSISTANT PRODUCTION MANAGER
T.A. Landis

COVER PHOTO
Jim Graham (photography)
Janice Engelke (art direction)

The clinical procedures described and recommended in this publication are based on research and consultation with medical and nursing authorities. To the best of our knowledge, these procedures reflect currently accepted clinical practice; nevertheless, they can't be considered absolute and universal recommendations. For individual application, treatment recommendations must be considered in light of the patient's clinical condition and, before administration of new or infrequently used drugs, in light of the latest package-insert information. The authors and the publisher disclaim responsibility for any adverse effects resulting directly or indirectly from the suggested procedures, from any undetected errors, or from the reader's misunderstanding of the text.

PBA-010687

ISBN 0-87434-122-1

Contents

Contributors

At the time of original publication, these contributors held the following positions.

Lynne Atkinson, RN, BSN, CEN. Formerly Emergency Medical Services Coordinator at Metropolitan Hospital, Parkview Division (Philadelphia), Ms. Atkinson earned her nursing degree at Holy Family College, Philadelphia. An Advanced Cardiac Life-Support Instructor, she's currently president of the Emergency Nurses' Association's Philadelphia chapter; she also belongs to the American Trauma Society.

Kay Bensing, RN, BS, MA, MJ. Currently a staff nurse at the Philadelphia Psychiatric Center, Ms. Bensing received her nursing education at the Reading (Pa.) Hospital School of Nursing and the Temple University Hospital School of Nursing (Philadelphia). She also holds graduate degrees in education from Loyola-Marymount University in Los Angeles and in journalism from Temple University.

Susan Babbitt DeJong, RN, BSN. Ms. DeJong, who received her BSN from Cornell University–New York Hospital School of Nursing in New York City, is currently a critical care consultant based in Wynnewood, Pa. She previously held the position of Head Nurse, Pediatric Intensive Care (isolation) at Children's Hospital of Philadelphia. Ms. DeJong belongs to the American Association of Critical-Care Nurses (AACN) and to the AACN's southeastern Pennsylvania chapter.

Joan E. Mason, RN, BS, EdM. A nurse consultant and clinical editor at Springhouse Corporation, Ms. Mason formerly held positions as Nursing Instructor at Philadelphia General Hospital School of Nursing and Staff Education Director at Roxborough Memorial Hospital (Philadelphia). She received her RN diploma from Temple University Hospital School of Nursing; she also holds graduate degrees in nursing education and health education from Temple University. A member of the Pennsylvania Nurses' Association, Ms. Mason serves on the American Nurses' Association's Council on Continuing Education, the steering committee of the Delaware Valley Inservice Association, and the advisory board for Professional Nursing Development. She also belongs to the American Association of Critical-Care Nurses.

Timothy O. Morgan, RN, CCRN. Mr. Morgan is Trauma Nurse Coordinator for the Southern New Jersey Regional Trauma Center in Camden, N.J. A graduate of Gloucester County College in Sewell, N.J., he belongs to the American Association of Critical-Care Nurses; Emergency Department Nurses Association; American Society for Testing and Materials, Subcommittee F-30 on Emergency Services; American Trauma Society; and Trauma Nurse Network.

Caring for the Emergency Patient

Basic life support	Shock and trauma care
Adult ACLS	Burn care
Pediatric ACLS	Digoxin overdose
Neonatal ACLS	

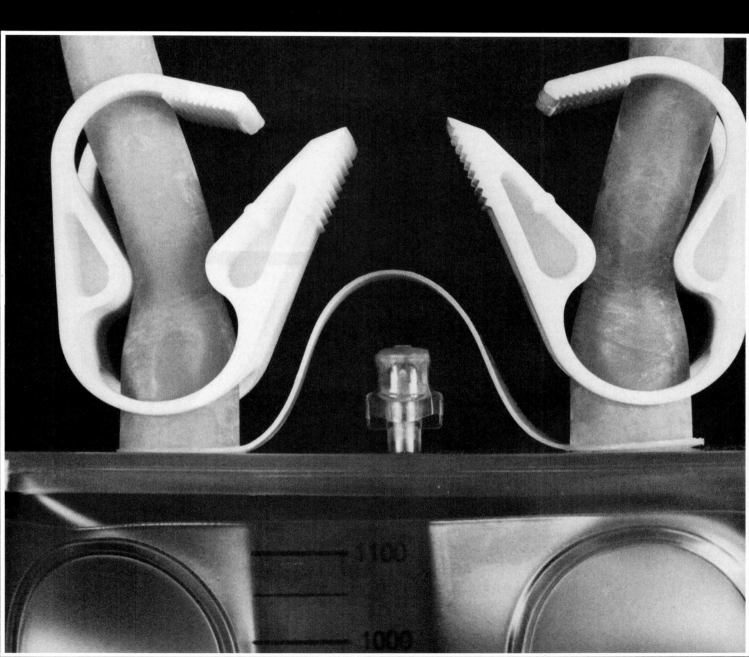

Basic life support

By definition, basic life support (BLS) either prevents respiratory or circulatory arrest (for example, by clearing an airway obstruction) or supports respiration and circulation postarrest with cardiopulmonary resuscitation (CPR). Advanced cardiac life support (ACLS), which we'll discuss beginning on page 14, augments BLS with emergency drugs and equipment.

The guidelines for BLS and ACLS presented in this PHOTOBOOK reflect American Heart Association standards published in 1986.* Use this information as an adjunct to life-support training and periodic refresher courses.

The photostories on the following pages reflect current CPR recommendations. Note that CPR procedures no longer differ for adults and children, with these exceptions: for most children (depending on size), seal both nose and mouth during artificial respiration, use only one hand for chest compressions, and compress only 1" to 1½" (compared to 1½" to 2" for adults).

* "Standards and Guidelines for Cardiopulmonary Resuscitation and Emergency Cardiac Care," *Journal of the American Medical Association* 255(21):2841-3044, June 6, 1986.

CPR and disease transmission: Safety considerations

Some health care workers who perform CPR frequently worry about the risk of contracting such diseases as hepatitis B and acquired immune deficiency syndrome (AIDS). To date, no case of hepatitis B transmitted during CPR has been documented; AIDS transmission via CPR seems similarly unlikely. However, because of a theoretical infection risk, the American Heart Association (AHA) suggests using disposable airway equipment or resuscitation bags and wearing gloves when in contact with blood and other body fluids. Clear plastic face masks with one-way valves, which direct the victim's exhalations away from the rescuer, may provide added protection during CPR.

Regarding similar concerns about manikin use during CPR training, the AHA notes that when outside the body, both hepatitis B and AIDS viruses succumb to disinfectant chemicals. The following precautions minimize risks:
• Students with AIDS, hepatitis, upper respiratory tract infections, or hand or mouth lesions shouldn't participate in training.
• Students should work in pairs, with each pair using only one manikin. Each student should demonstrate good hygiene— for example, by hand washing before manikin contact.
• Individual protective face shields, if used, should be changed between contacts by different students. Between contacts (including finger sweeps), the manikin's face and airway should be wiped vigorously with dry gauze, then wetted with either sodium hypochlorite or 70% alcohol. Allow surfaces to remain wet for at least 30 seconds; then dry them with clean gauze.
• During two-person CPR training, when the manikin can't be disinfected between students, the second student should simulate ventilation, rather than blow into the manikin airway.
• Manikins should be scrubbed and disinfected with sodium hypochlorite after training sessions, according to the manufacturer's specifications. They should also be routinely inspected for cracks, which harbor microbes.

How to open an airway: Two techniques

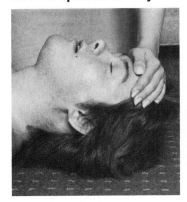

1 Currently recommended to open an airway under most circumstances, the *head-tilt/chin-lift maneuver* works more effectively than the previously recommended head-tilt/neck-lift maneuver.

To begin, place one hand on the victim's forehead and tilt the head back by applying firm backward pressure with the palm, as shown.

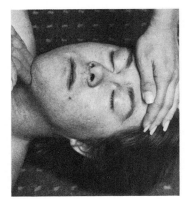

2 Then put the fingers (not the thumb) of your other hand under the lower jaw's bony portion (near the chin) and bring the chin forward. (Don't press too hard under the chin, or you may obstruct the airway.) Take care not to close the mouth completely (unless you're performing mouth-to-nose respiration). Remove dentures if they interfere with positioning.

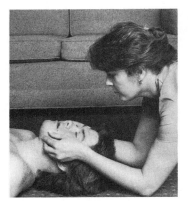

3 Although more difficult to perform than the head-tilt/chin-lift maneuver, the *jaw-thrust maneuver* can open the airway without hyperextending the neck. Try it first if you suspect a cervical spine injury. Rest your elbows on the surface supporting the victim's head and place a hand on each side of his lower jaw, at its angles.

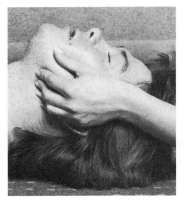

4 Lift with both hands to displace the mandible forward while tilting the head backward. Support the head, so it doesn't tilt backward or turn to the side. If the lips close, retract them with your thumb. Before giving mouth-to-mouth respiration, block the nostrils with your cheek. *Note:* If these steps don't open the airway, tilt the head backward very slightly.

UPDATE

BLS standards: How they've changed

Here's a quick look at how current basic life-support (BLS) standards compare to previous standards.

Current standard	Previous standard	Rationale for change
• Use the head-tilt/chin-lift method to open the airway.	• The head-tilt/neck-lift method was recommended for opening the airway.	• The head-tilt/chin-lift method opens the airway more effectively. (*Note:* Use the jaw thrust or chin lift without the head-tilt maneuver if you suspect a cervical spine injury.)
• Give two initial breaths (1 to 1½ seconds/breath) when attempting to ventilate. (Pause to inhale between breaths.)	• Four quick breaths, with no pause between breaths, were recommended.	• Two breaths reduce the risk of gastric distention, regurgitation, and aspiration.
• When giving chest compressions during two-rescuer CPR, pause after every fifth compression so your partner can deliver one ventilation lasting 1 to 1½ seconds.	• During two-rescuer CPR, chest compressions continued during ventilation. A breath was delivered on the upstroke of the fifth compression.	• This change also reduces the risk of gastric distention.
• Deliver 80 to 100 compressions/minute when doing either one- or two-rescuer adult CPR.	• During two-rescuer adult CPR, the recommended rate was 60 to 80 compressions/minute. (The 80 to 100 compressions/minute recommended for one-rescuer adult or child CPR remains the same.)	• By increasing intrathoracic pressure, the faster rate promotes better blood flow to the heart and brain.
• After opening an infant's airway, deliver two gentle breaths (1 to 1½ seconds/breath); pause between breaths.	• Four quick, gentle breaths were recommended, with no pause between breaths.	• As in adults, this change reduces the risk of gastric distention, regurgitation, and aspiration.
• On an infant, perform chest compressions one fingerbreadth below the nipple line.	• Chest compressions were performed at the nipple line.	• Recent studies reveal that an infant's heart lies slightly lower in the chest than previously thought.
• When performing the Heimlich maneuver on an adult, *do not* deliver back blows. Deliver abdominal thrusts only (or chest thrusts for an obese or pregnant victim).	• Four initial back blows were recommended for adults.	• Back blows may be ineffective and even dangerous for an adult. (Continue to use back blows and chest thrusts for an infant under age 1.)

Positioning your hands for chest compressions: A review

Before beginning chest compressions, position your hands at the correct location, as shown below. Follow these steps:
• With the middle and index fingers of the hand closer to the victim's legs, locate the rib cage's lower margin.
• Next, run these two fingers up the rib cage to the notch where the ribs meet the sternum.
• Put your middle finger on this notch, and place your index finger next to it. Then place the heel of your opposite hand next to the index finger, on the long axis of the sternum. (See first illustration.)
• Now place your first hand on top of the other, so both hands are parallel and the fingers point away from you. Extend or interlace your fingers, and begin compressions. (See second illustration.)

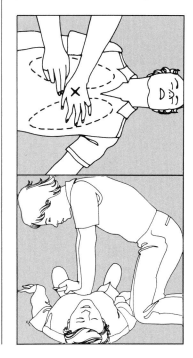

Basic life support

How to activate the EMS system

You're visiting a neighbor when he suffers cardiac arrest. Can you quickly activate the emergency medical services (EMS) system? Follow these guidelines.

If you're alone, perform CPR for about 1 minute; then call your local emergency number (for example, 911). Be prepared to give concise, accurate information, including:
- where the emergency occurred (with cross streets, if possible)
- the number of the telephone closest to the emergency site
- what happened (for example, the victim had a heart attack or was struck by a car)
- the victim's condition
- what aid he's receiving
- how many people need help.

If you can't activate the EMS system, continue one-rescuer CPR.

How cough CPR combats ventricular dysrhythmias

Continuous, forceful coughs spaced 1 to 3 seconds apart may help convert potentially lethal ventricular tachycardia or fibrillation into a normal sinus rhythm—or at least may buy the patient time until other emergency measures take effect. Coughing closes the epiglottis and causes respiratory muscles to contract forcefully. As the illustrations below show, increased intrathoracic pressure propels blood forward, maintaining cerebral and myocardial perfusion. Consequently, the patient remains conscious.

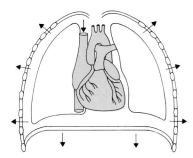

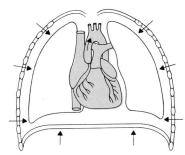

A deep breath lowers intrathoracic pressure, promoting venous return to the heart.

A deep cough raises intrathoracic pressure. Increased aortic pressure and reflex coronary vasodilation secondary to baroreceptor activation contribute to improved myocardial perfusion.

Performing CPR

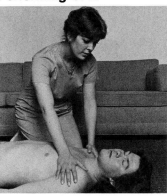

1 If you discover someone who's unconscious, first determine unresponsiveness by tapping or gently shaking his shoulder and shouting, "Are you OK?" Then call for help.

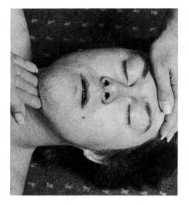

2 If necessary, turn him onto his back. Move his body as a unit, supporting his head and neck. (If he's in bed, place a backboard under him.) Then open his airway, using the head-tilt/chin-lift maneuver. *Caution:* Use a chin-lift or jaw-thrust maneuver *without* head-tilt if you suspect a cervical spine injury.

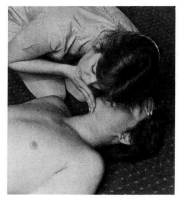

3 Now, determine breathlessness. While maintaining the open airway, place your ear over the victim's mouth and watch his chest. Look, listen, and feel for breathing for 3 to 5 seconds.

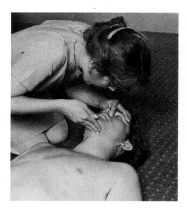

4 After you establish that the victim's not breathing, seal his mouth and nose and ventilate twice (1 to 1½ seconds for each ventilation). Watch for his chest to rise, which indicates adequate ventilation volume. *Important:* Allow time for the chest to deflate between ventilations.

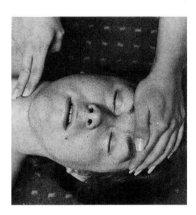

5 Next, determine pulselessness by feeling for the carotid pulse on the side nearer to you. Check for 5 to 10 seconds while maintaining the open airway.

If someone responded to your call for help, send him to activate the emergency medical services system.

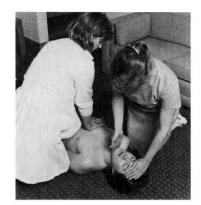

9 Resume the head-tilt/chin-lift maneuver to open the airway. Deliver one ventilation; the second rescuer then delivers five compressions in 3 to 4 seconds (compression rate: 80 to 100/minute). Continue ventilating the victim once for every 5 compressions. To maintain rhythm, the second rescuer should say, "One-and-two-and-three-and-four-and-five, pause, vent."

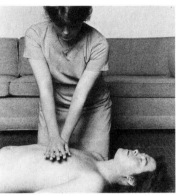

6 To begin chest compressions, check landmarks and position your hands properly. Compress the victim's sternum 1½" to 2". During the upstroke, keep your hands in position on the sternum and allow the chest to relax. Deliver four cycles of 15 compressions (compressing and relaxing evenly) and 2 ventilations (compression rate: 80 to 100/minute; ventilation duration: 1 to 1½ seconds each).

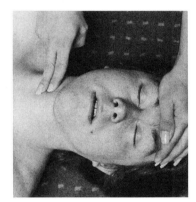

10 Between ventilations, check the victim's pulse to determine compression effectiveness. Deliver at least 10 compression/ventilation cycles.

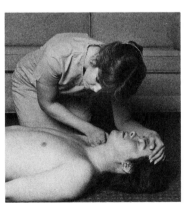

7 Check for pulse and spontaneous breathing. If they don't return, resume by delivering 2 ventilations and 15 compressions; deliver four such ventilation/compression cycles.

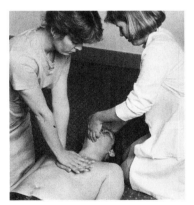

11 When the second rescuer tires, she should say, "Change-one-and-two-and-three-and-four-and-five." Immediately after the ventilation, both rescuers change position simultaneously.

The second rescuer now opens the airway, as shown here.

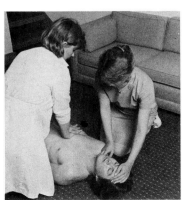

8 If a second rescuer arrives, she should announce that she knows CPR and get into position to deliver chest compressions. Complete the ventilation/compression cycle and check for pulse and breathing.

If you don't detect a pulse or breathing, say, "No pulse. Continue CPR."

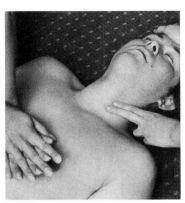

12 The second rescuer also performs a 5-second pulse check. If she fails to detect a pulse, she says, "No pulse. Continue CPR." Then she delivers one ventilation. Resume compression/ventilation cycles.

Basic life support

Clearing an obstructed airway

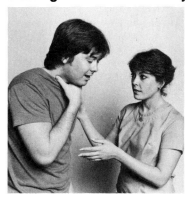

1 To help someone who appears to be choking, first determine if he can speak by asking, "Are you choking?" If he can speak, cough, or breathe, stand by but don't intervene.

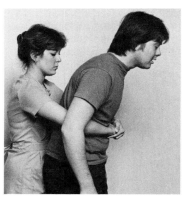

2 If he can't speak, cough, or breathe, perform abdominal thrusts (the Heimlich maneuver): stand behind him, wrap your arms around his waist, and place the thumb side of one fist against his abdomen at midline (slightly above the navel; well below the xyphoid tip). Grasp the fist with your other hand and make quick upward thrusts. Repeat until you're successful or the victim loses consciousness.

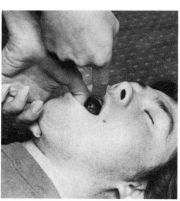

3 If he becomes unconscious, position him supine and call for help (or activate the emergency medical services system). Open his mouth with a tongue-jaw lift and sweep deeply into his mouth with your finger (finger sweep). *Caution:* If the victim's a child, do the finger-sweep maneuver *only* if you can see a foreign object.

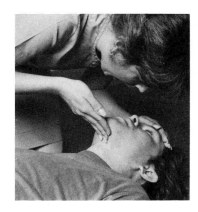

4 Open his airway with the head-tilt/chin-lift maneuver, and attempt to ventilate.

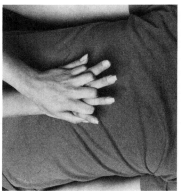

5 If you don't succeed, straddle the victim's thighs and position the heel of one hand against his abdomen at the midline point described in Step 2 at left. Place your other hand on top of it, as shown here, and deliver 6 to 10 abdominal thrusts. *Note:* Use chest thrusts for obese victims and women in the late stages of pregnancy.

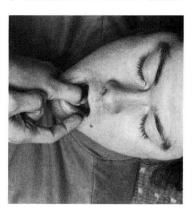

6 Open the victim's mouth and perform a finger sweep. (If the victim's a child, do this step *only* if you can see the object.) Then open his airway with the head-tilt/chin-lift maneuver, and attempt to ventilate. If unsuccessful, repeat the procedure as necessary.

AT THE SCENE

Airway obstruction: Cause unknown

If you find a victim who's unconscious for unknown reasons, the rescue procedure differs slightly from the procedure outlined in the previous photostory. Follow these steps:
• Determine unresponsiveness by tapping or shaking his shoulder and shouting, "Are you OK?" Then call for help.
• Position him supine and open his airway with the head-tilt/chin-lift maneuver.
• Look, listen, and feel for breathing for 3 to 5 seconds.
• If he's not breathing, attempt to ventilate. If you can't, re-

position his head and try again.
• If you're still unsuccessful, activate the emergency medical services system.
• Straddle the victim and perform 6 to 10 abdominal thrusts (see step 5 above).
• Use the tongue-jaw lift to open his mouth. Perform a deep finger sweep to remove a foreign body, if present.
• Open his airway and attempt to ventilate. If you're unsuccessful, repeat the procedure as necessary.

Performing infant CPR

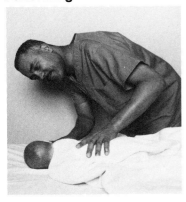

1 Modify basic CPR techniques for an infant, using the guidelines shown here. For demonstration purposes, we're using a Resusci-Baby in this and the following photostory.
Determine unresponsiveness by tapping or gently shaking the infant's shoulder.

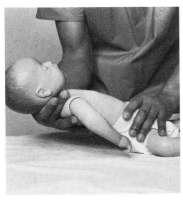

2 Then turn him on his back as a unit, supporting his head and neck. Make sure he's on a hard surface.

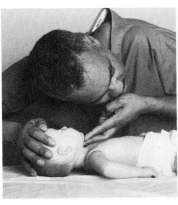

3 Use the head-tilt/chin-lift maneuver to position his head in a neutral or sniffing position. *Don't hyperextend his neck.*

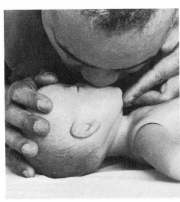

4 After determining breathlessness, seal his nose and mouth with your mouth and ventilate twice.

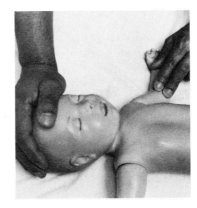

5 Determine pulselessness by feeling for the brachial pulse. Maintain the head tilt with your other hand, as the nurse is doing here.

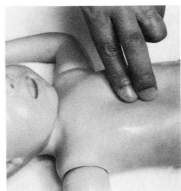

6 To position your fingers for chest compressions, draw an imaginary line between the infant's nipples. Then place two or three fingers on his sternum, one finger's width below the imaginary line.

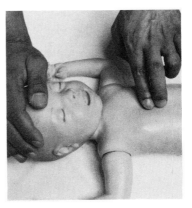

7 Compress vertically ½" to 1". Keep your fingers on the sternum during the upstroke. Keep compression and relaxation times equal. Maintain a compression rate of at least 100/minute (5 compressions in 3 seconds or less).

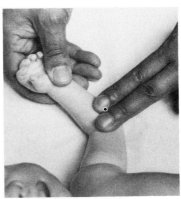

8 Perform 10 cycles of 5 compressions and 1 ventilation. Use this mnemonic: one-two-three-four-five-pause-head tilt-chin lift-ventilate-continue compressions. After 10 cycles, check the brachial pulse to determine pulselessness.

Basic life support

Clearing an infant's airway

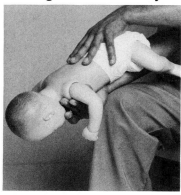

1 If a conscious infant appears to be choking, assess his condition by looking, listening, and feeling for breathing. Observe for blue lips.

To clear an obstruction, support his head and neck by holding his jaw with one hand. Position him over your arm, with his head lower than his trunk, as shown here. Use your thigh to support your forearm.

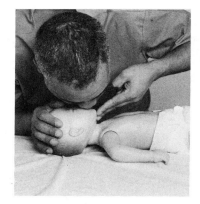

5 If the infant becomes unconscious, call for help and activate the emergency medical services system. Then open the airway with a tongue-jaw lift and look for the foreign body. Attempt to remove it *only if you can see it.*

Open the infant's airway with a head-tilt/chin-lift maneuver and attempt to ventilate, as shown.

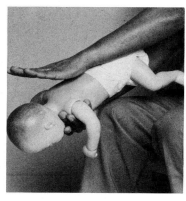

2 Deliver four forceful back blows between the shoulder blades with the heel of your hand.

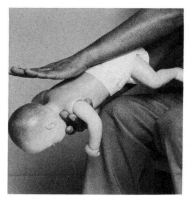

6 If you can't ventilate the infant, position him head-down, as shown, and deliver four back blows.

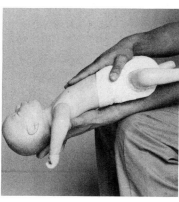

3 Next, sandwich the infant between your hands and turn him on his back, head lower than trunk. Continue to support his head throughout.

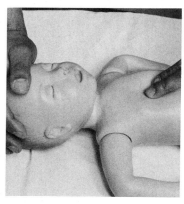

7 Then turn the infant and deliver four chest thrusts.

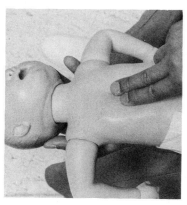

4 Deliver four chest thrusts in the midsternal region. Use the same technique you'd use to deliver chest compressions (see page 11), but deliver the thrusts at a slower rate.

Repeat back blows and chest thrusts until you dislodge the foreign object or the infant loses consciousness.

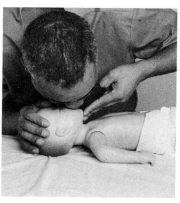

8 Open the airway with a tongue-jaw lift, and look for the foreign body. Attempt to remove it only if you can see it. Then open the airway with a head-tilt/chin-lift maneuver and attempt to ventilate, as shown.

Repeat the sequence until it's effective.

Applying rescue techniques under special circumstances

Some emergency situations require you to modify life-support techniques. Consider these examples:

Traumatic injury
A victim of cardiac arrest from traumatic injury may respond poorly to external chest compression, particularly if he's hypovolemic. Assess the ABCs (airway, breathing, and circulation), begin appropriate treatment (including hemorrhage control with direct pressure, as needed), and transport him to a trauma center as quickly as possible. *Note:* A victim with severe facial injuries may need a cricothyroidotomy.

Protect the cervical spine. If you suspect cervical spine fracture, avoid turning or tilting the head. To turn the patient, support his head, neck, chest, and abdomen, and turn his body as a unit. Open the airway with a jaw-thrust or a chin-lift maneuver *without* head-tilt.

Electric shock
When attempting a rescue, first make sure you won't endanger yourself by touching the victim. Move him away from the electrical source, and assess him for breathing and circulation. Begin CPR, as indicated. Also assess for related injuries requiring immediate attention, for example, burns and traumatic injury from a fall.

Electric shock can cause these conditions:
• tetany of breathing muscles (This usually lasts only during exposure to current; however, prolonged exposure may trigger cardiac arrest from hypoxia.)
• prolonged breathing muscle paralysis
• ventricular fibrillation or asystole.

Note: Because lightning depolarizes the entire myocardium simultaneously, normal sinus rhythm may resume spontaneously. Lightning victims who don't suffer immediate cardiac arrest have a high survival rate.

Near drowning
Initiate mouth-to-mouth or mouth-to-nose respiration as soon as possible—while the victim's still in the water, if possible. Unless an obstruction exists, don't attempt to expel water from the airway first—most drowning victims inhale relatively little water. Attempting to remove it by any means except suction may cause the victim to aspirate stomach contents. Administer abdominal thrusts (the Heimlich maneuver) only if clearly indicated.

Don't attempt chest compressions in the water (unless you have special training), because they'll be ineffective without a rigid back support.

If you suspect injury to the cervical spine, support the victim's neck in a neutral position and float him supine onto a firm surface (such as a surfboard) before removing him from the water. Use the precautions discussed above *(Traumatic injury)* for turning and providing artificial respiration.

Transport the victim to an advanced life-support facility as soon as possible, even if he revived quickly. *Note:* Many near-drowning victims recover fully from prolonged submersion in very cold water. Always treat such a victim aggressively unless you see tissue decay or other obvious signs of death. Read what follows for more on treating hypothermia.

Hypothermia
Brain function depression and vasoconstriction obscure vital signs in victims of severe hypothermia (body temperature below 86° F., or 30° C.). Begin artificial respiration, as indicated. Take up to a minute to check for pulse (the patient may have extreme bradycardia); then begin chest compressions if indicated. Prevent further heat loss by wrapping the victim and applying warmth externally—for example, with warm packs or warm moist oxygen. *Caution:* Keep the patient still and perform only essential procedures—excessive movement can trigger ventricular fibrillation. Defibrillation shocks may not be effective in severe hypothermia.

If the victim receives emergency drugs, adjust the dosage as ordered and monitor him closely for toxicity—hypothermia reduces drug metabolism.

To reduce the risk of rewarming shock, help to rewarm the victim's core. Techniques include heated, humidified ventilation; peritoneal dialysis; thoracotomy; and extracorporeal blood warming with partial bypass.

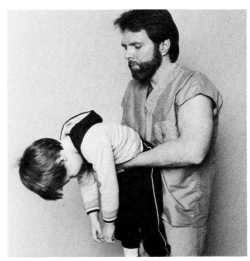

Clearing a child's airway
To help a conscious child with an airway obstruction, the American Heart Association now recommends the Heimlich maneuver (see page 10). Lift a small child, as shown here.

BLS certification: New standards
Basic life-support (BLS) training and certification now fall into the following five categories. Certification cards, valid for up to 2 years, indicate courses successfully completed, instead of the previous levels of certification. (The American Heart Association encourages cardholders to recertify more frequently than once every 2 years.)
• *BLS Course A:* Heartsaver and adult obstructed airway. (Most laymen take this course.)
• *BLS Course B:* Course A plus pediatric CPR. (Laymen with a specific interest in pediatric CPR—for example, parents with a child who may need resuscitation—take this course.)
• *BLS Course C:* Heartsaver, adult and pediatric obstructed airway, and pediatric one-rescuer and two-rescuer CPR. (Previously called Basic Rescuer Certification, this course remains appropriate for health care professionals and other professional rescuers.)
• *BLS Course D:* Pediatric obstructed airway and CPR.
• *BLS Course E:* Instruction designed for rescuers with special concerns or problems, for example, handicapped rescuers.

Adult ACLS

Provided by emergency facilities and mobile emergency units, advanced cardiac life support (ACLS) includes basic life support, which we discussed in the preceding pages. As defined by the American Heart Association, ACLS also includes these components:
- adjunctive equipment and special techniques for maintaining circulation and ventilation
- electrocardiogram monitoring
- intravenous access
- drug and electrical therapies (for example, defibrillation) to combat cardiac and respiratory arrest and to stabilize the patient postarrest
- treatment for acute myocardial infarction.

In the following pages, we'll focus on updated standards in these areas. *Remember:* Like BLS, ACLS requires hands-on training and periodic refresher courses. Use this information as an adjunct only.

Drug therapy guidelines

Top priorities in advanced life support include oxygen, I.V. fluid administration, and drug administration. In acute myocardial infarction (AMI), you'll also provide pain relief.

Oxygen therapy. Give 100% oxygen (or the highest concentration available). When given with ventilation and circulatory support, oxygen therapy improves arterial oxygen tension, hemoglobin saturation, and tissue oxygenation.

I.V. therapy. Establish an I.V. line as quickly as possible. Drugs take effect faster when given through a large central vein (rather than a peripheral vein), but establishing a central line interrupts CPR.

Drugs given via a peripheral vein need about 2 minutes to reach the central circulation. Administering large volumes of flush solution and elevating extremities may also help move drugs into the central circulation quickly.

In the absence of venous access, you can give many drugs (including epinephrine, lidocaine, and atropine) endotracheally. The doctor gives epinephrine by intracardiac injection only if venous and endotracheal routes aren't available.

Besides drug administration, use an I.V. line to administer fluids, if indicated—expanding circulating blood volume combats severe blood loss. Volume expansion fluids include whole blood, Ringer's solution, 0.9% saline solution, and colloid solutions. Keep I.V. lines open with dextrose 5% in water.

Pain relief. As ordered, give morphine sulfate to counter AMI pain. In addition to relieving pain and anxiety, morphine helps decrease myocardial oxygen demand by decreasing venous return and inducing moderate arterial vasodilation. To reduce the risk of respiratory depression and hypotension in a volume-depleted patient, give morphine in small I.V. doses (2 to 5 mg), as ordered.

Read the following chart for current recommendations on specific ACLS drugs.

ACLS drug update

Most of the drugs in this chart act either to control heart rhythm and rate, or to improve cardiac output and blood pressure through peripheral vasoconstriction and inotropic or chronotropic cardiac effects. (For a discussion of beta blockers and diuretics, which don't appear in this chart, see page 17.)

Amrinone lactate

A nonadrenergic cardiotonic agent that causes vasodilation and increases cardiac function

Indication
- Congestive heart failure

Dosage and administration
Give one 0.75-mg/kg dose I.V. over 2 to 3 minutes, followed by 5 to 10 mcg/kg/min I.V. infusion.

Special considerations
- Amrinone may exacerbate myocardial ischemia in dosages greater than 20 mcg/kg/min.

Atropine sulfate

A parasympatholytic agent that reduces cardiac vagal tone, enhances sinus node discharge rate, and improves atrioventricular (AV) conduction

Indications
- Sinus bradycardia with hemodynamic compromise (for example, hypotension)
- Sinus bradycardia with frequent ventricular ectopic beats
- Ventricular asystole

Dosage and administration
For bradycardia: 0.5 mg I.V. every 5 minutes, to a total of 2 mg.
For asystole: 1 mg I.V.; repeat after 5 minutes if asystole persists.

Special considerations
- Atropine may be given endotracheally.
- Dosages below 0.5 mg have parasympathomimetic effects and therefore may slow heart rate.
- Use cautiously in acute myocardial ischemia or infarction; excessive rate increases may widen areas of ischemia or infarction.
- Monitor for ventricular tachycardia or fibrillation (rare complications).

Bretylium tosylate

An antiarrhythmic that initially exerts transient adrenergic stimulation, followed by adrenergic blocking

Indications
- Resistant ventricular tachycardia or fibrillation

Dosage and administration
For resistant ventricular tachycardia: 5 to 10 mg/kg diluted to 50 ml with dextrose 5% in water (D_5W) and injected I.V. over 8 to 10 minutes. Follow loading dose with a continuous I.V. infusion at 1 to 2 mg/min.
For resistant ventricular fibrillation: 5 mg/kg I.V. bolus followed by defibrillation. If indicated, increase dose to 10 mg/kg and give at 15- to 30-minute intervals, to a maximum of 30 mg/kg.

Special considerations
• Don't use as a first-line drug. Use only if lidocaine and defibrillation fail to convert ventricular fibrillation, if lidocaine fails to prevent ventricular fibrillation from recurring, or if lidocaine and procainamide fail to control ventricular tachycardia associated with pulse.

Calcium salts

A critical electrolyte that aids myocardial contraction and impulse formation

Indications
• Not recommended for routine use during resuscitation efforts. However, calcium may be ordered to improve myocardial contractility when hyperkalemia, hypocalcemia, or calcium channel blocker drug toxicity also exists.

Dosage and administration
Give 2 ml of a 10% solution of calcium chloride (2 to 4 mg/kg); repeat as ordered. Administer calcium gluceptate in a 5- to 7-ml dose; calcium gluconate, in a 5- to 8-ml dose.

Special considerations
• Current research supports using calcium only for the specific conditions listed above. Calcium hasn't proved effective in treating cardiac arrest in all situations; in any cardiac emergency, high calcium levels induced by calcium administration may be detrimental.

Dobutamine hydrochloride

A synthetic catecholamine primarily stimulating beta-receptors; a potent inotropic agent

Indication
• Heart failure

Dosage and administration
Give 2.5 to 10 mcg/kg/min I.V.

Special considerations
• Dobutamine may induce reflex peripheral vasodilation.
• As ordered, give with sodium nitroprusside for synergistic effect.
• Monitor heart rate closely. An increase of 10% or more may exacerbate myocardial ischemia (a common problem at dosages above 20 mcg/kg/min).

Dopamine hydrochloride

A chemical precursor of norepinephrine; stimulates alpha-, beta-, and dopaminergic receptors. Effects vary with dosage.

Indication
• Shock

Dosage and administration
Give 2 to 5 mcg/kg/min I.V. initially and titrate according to response.

Special considerations
• At low dosages (1 to 2 mcg/kg/min), dopamine dilates renal and mesenteric vessels without increasing heart rate or blood pressure. At higher dosages (2 to 10 mcg/kg/min), it primarily stimulates beta-receptors, increasing cardiac output without peripheral vasoconstriction. At dosages above 10 mcg/kg/min, it stimulates alpha-receptors, causing peripheral vasoconstriction.
• Don't give dopamine in same I.V. line as sodium bicarbonate. The alkaline solution may inactivate dopamine.

Epinephrine hydrochloride

A naturally occurring catecholamine with alpha-adrenergic stimulating effects; a first-line drug for treating cardiac arrest

Indication
• Cardiac arrest

Dosage and administration
Give 0.5 to 1 mg (5 to 10 ml of a 1:10,000 solution) I.V. or 1 mg (10 ml of a 1:10,000 solution) endotracheally. Repeat every 5 minutes during resuscitation efforts.

Special considerations
• Intracardiac injection is contraindicated unless venous and endotracheal routes are unavailable. Intracardiac injection interrupts resuscitation efforts and risks such complications as coronary artery laceration, cardiac tamponade, and pneumothorax.
• Don't give in same I.V. line as sodium bicarbonate or any other alkaline solution.

Isoproterenol hydrochloride

A synthetic sympathomimetic with exclusively beta-adrenergic stimulating effects

Indication
• Hemodynamically significant bradycardia unresponsive to atropine, in a patient with a pulse

Dosage and administration
Add 1 mg isoproterenol to 500 ml of D_5W. Give 2 to 10 mcg/min I.V. infusion. Titrate according to patient response.

Special considerations
• Isoproterenol is not indicated in cardiac arrest.
• Isoproterenol's potent inotropic and chronotropic effects increase cardiac output and work load, exacerbating ischemia and dysrhythmias in patients with ischemic heart disease.
• Use this drug only as a temporary measure until pacemaker therapy begins.

Lidocaine

The drug of choice for ventricular dysrhythmias

Indications
• Ventricular tachycardia
• Ventricular fibrillation
• Premature ventricular contractions (PVCs) that are frequent, close-coupled, multiform in configuration, or arranged in short bursts of two or more in succession
• Myocardial infarction (to prevent ventricular fibrillation)

Dosage and administration
Give 1 mg/kg I.V. bolus, followed by 0.5-mg/kg boluses every 8 to 10 minutes, as necessary, to a total of 3 mg/kg.

Adult ACLS

ACLS drug update continued

Lidocaine continued

Special considerations
• Lidocaine may be used prophylactically when myocardial infarction is suspected but not confirmed.
• In ventricular fibrillation, lidocaine improves response to defibrillation.
• Give only bolus doses during resuscitation efforts. After resuscitation, give a continuous infusion at 2 to 4 mg/min. (Reduce dosage and monitor drug blood levels after 24 hours, as ordered.)
• In emergencies that don't require resuscitation, follow the initial bolus with a continuous infusion, as ordered.

Nitroglycerin

A vascular smooth muscle relaxant

Indications
• Congestive heart failure
• Unstable angina

Dosage and administration
Give 10 mcg/min I.V. Increase in increments of 5 to 10 mcg/min, as needed.

Special considerations
• Most patients respond to 200 mcg/min or less. Mean dosage range: 50 to 500 mcg/min.
• Monitor for hypotension, a side effect that exacerbates myocardial ischemia.

Norepinephrine

A naturally occurring catecholamine with both beta-adrenergic stimulating effects (improved cardiac contractility) and alpha-adrenergic stimulating effects (vasoconstriction)

Indications
• Severe hypotension with low total peripheral resistance

Dosage and administration
Add 4 or 8 mg norepinephrine injection to 500 ml of D_5W or dextrose 5% in normal saline solution. Administer the resulting concentration (8 and 16 mcg/ml, respectively) I.V., titrating according to patient response.

Special considerations
• Norepinephrine is contraindicated in hypovolemia.
• Cardiac output may increase or decrease following norepinephrine administration, depending on vascular resistance, the left ventricle's ability to function, and reflex responses.
• Don't give in same I.V. line as alkaline solutions.
• Monitor blood pressure with an intraarterial line, because standard blood pressure measurements may be falsely low.

Procainamide hydrochloride

An antiarrhythmic that depresses the myocardium by exerting both a direct and indirect (anticholinergic) effect

Indications
• Ventricular dysrhythmias, such as PVCs or tachycardia, when lidocaine is contraindicated or ineffective

Dosage and administration
In an emergency, give 20 mg/min up to a total dose of 1 g. Usual dosage: 50 mg I.V. every 5 minutes until desired response is achieved, up to a total of 1 g. Maintenance infusion rate: 1 to 4 mg/min.

Special considerations
• Reduce dosage in patients with renal failure.
• Guard against too-rapid infusion, which causes acute hypotension. Use particular caution in patients with acute myocardial infarction.
• Monitor for widening QRS complex. If QRS complex widens more than 50%, notify doctor and discontinue infusion, as ordered.

Sodium bicarbonate

An electrolyte solution used to maintain acid-base balance

Indications
• Not recommended for use during initial resuscitation efforts (unless preexisting acidosis is clearly present). May be used at team leader's discretion after such interventions as defibrillation, cardiac compression, and administration of first-line drugs.

Dosage and administration
Give 1 mEq/kg initially, followed by no more than half this dose every 10 minutes thereafter. Postresuscitation, give sodium bicarbonate, as indicated by arterial blood gas measurements.

Special considerations
• Consider hyperventilation, not sodium bicarbonate, the primary therapy for controlling acid-base balance.

Sodium nitroprusside

A fast-acting peripheral vasodilator that decreases peripheral arterial resistance. May improve cardiac output without causing great changes in systemic blood pressure or heart rate.

Indications
• Heart failure
• Hypertensive crisis

Dosage and administration
Add 50 mg to 250 to 1,000 ml of D_5W. Initially give 10 to 20 mcg/min.

Special considerations
• Wrap drug container in opaque material—light causes drug deterioration. (You needn't wrap I.V. tubing, however.)

Verapamil hydrochloride

A calcium channel blocker that dilates coronary arteries and reduces cardiac oxygen demand by decreasing systemic vascular resistance (afterload). Also depresses SA and AV nodal conduction.

Indications
• Atrial dysrhythmias, especially paroxysmal supraventricular tachycardias (PSVTs) with AV node conduction

Dosage and administration
Give 5 mg I.V. initially, followed by 10 mg in 15 to 30 minutes if dysrhythmia persists and patient hasn't responded adversely to initial dose.

Special considerations
• Monitor patient for hypotension, severe bradycardia, congestive heart failure, and facilitated accessory conduction in patients with Wolff-Parkinson-White syndrome.

Beta blockers and diuretics

In ACLS, beta blockers (such as propranolol hydrochloride) and diuretics (such as furosemide) help keep some patients stable after resuscitation. By blocking beta-receptors in the heart, beta blockers can help control recurring supraventricular tachycardias; they may also control some malignant ventricular dysrhythmias. Beta-blocker administration following cardiac arrest requires caution, however; these drugs can exacerbate heart failure. Also exercise caution in patients who depend on beta-adrenergic stimulation for hemodynamic stability and in those with asthma or heart failure.

Furosemide inhibits sodium reabsorption, mainly at the ascending loop of Henle. It may also have vascular effects: in patients with acute pulmonary edema, it may act as a venodilator; in those with chronic heart failure, it has transient vasoconstrictive effects. Vascular effects appear within 5 minutes of I.V. administration; diuresis takes longer. Use furosemide to treat cerebral edema and acute pulmonary edema after cardiac arrest.

Using the endotracheal route

If an I.V. line can't be established quickly in an emergency, the endotracheal (ET) tube offers an alternate access route for several first-line emergency drugs: epinephrine hydrochloride, atropine sulfate, and lidocaine hydrochloride. Once in the lungs, drugs pass through the alveoli and into the circulation. (Other drugs you can give by ET tube include naloxone hydrochloride and meta-raminol bitartrate.)

ET administration has distinct advantages over intracardiac injection, which interrupts resuscitation efforts and risks such complications as coronary artery laceration, cardiac tamponade, and pneumothorax. Current guidelines recommend intracardiac injection only as a last resort, when I.V. and endotracheal routes aren't available.

Onset of action varies according to such factors as the patient's hemodynamic status. Duration of action, however, typically lasts longer with ET administration owing to sustained absorption by the alveoli—a phenomenon called the *depot effect*. Consequently, you may need to adjust repeat doses and continuous infusions to prevent adverse drug effects.

Give the same initial drug dose through an ET tube that you'd give through a peripheral I.V. line. Dilute the dose to 5 to 10 ml to enhance absorption—with greater volume, a larger proportion of drug leaves the ET tube and contacts lung tissue. Use sterile water or normal saline solution as a diluent.

For details on the administration procedure, see the following photostory. *Caution:* Don't give these drugs by the ET route: bretylium, calcium, diazepam, isoproterenol, norepinephrine, and sodium bicarbonate.

Giving a drug through an ET tube

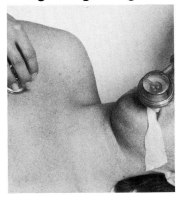

1 Prepare the medication. If a prefilled syringe isn't available, use a standard 5-ml or 10-ml syringe with needle or catheter securely attached. (Use the longest needle or catheter available so you can inject the drug deeply.)

Check ET tube placement, as the nurse is doing here. Make sure the patient's supine, with his head level with or slightly higher than his trunk.

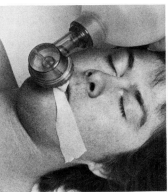

2 Quickly compress a positive-pressure oxygen delivery device (such as an Ambu bag) three to five times; then remove the device.

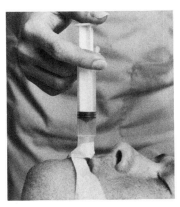

3 Inject the drug deep into the ET tube.

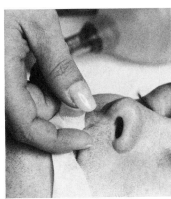

4 To prevent medication reflux, briefly place your thumb over the tube's opening, as shown here. Then reattach the Ambu bag and quickly compress it five times to distribute the medication and oxygenate the patient.

Monitor patient response. Onset of action may be quicker than you'd expect following peripheral I.V. administration. If the patient doesn't respond quickly, the doctor may order a repeat dose.

Adult ACLS

Defibrillation and cardioversion update

If initiated promptly, electrical therapy (defibrillation and cardioversion) can convert life-threatening dysrhythmias to normal cardiac rhythm. The following information reflects current ACLS guidelines.

Paddle size and placement

Use paddles 10 cm in diameter for most adults, 8 cm for older children, and 4.5 cm for infants. (For pediatric defibrillation and cardioversion guidelines, see page 23.)

To maximize current flow through the myocardium, place one paddle just to the right of the upper sternum and below the clavicle. Place the other to the left of the nipple, with its center in the midaxillary line (see illustration below, left). Or, as an alternative, place one paddle anteriorly over the left precordium; then place a special posterior paddle behind the heart (see illustration below, right). Apply about 25 lb pressure. *Caution:* If the patient has a permanent pacemaker, avoid placing a paddle within 5" of the pacemaker generator.

Energy level

Electrical current must be powerful enough to restore normal rhythm without damaging the heart or triggering another deadly dysrhythmia (for example, without converting ventricular tachycardia to ventricular fibrillation).

To defibrillate: For an adult in ventricular fibrillation, the first shock should be about 200 joules. Current standards recommend a second shock (if necessary) of 200 to 300 joules. If the second shock fails to defibrillate, immediately deliver a third shock not to exceed 360 joules. *Important:* For open-heart defibrillation, give only 5 joules for the initial shock and no more than 50 joules for any subsequent shock.

Begin defibrillation as soon as the equipment's available, even if you must interrupt basic life-support procedures to do so. Administer shocks rapidly, without interruption if possible. (Some older defibrillators take more than 30 seconds to recharge; some automatic defibrillators need up to 90 seconds to diagnose a dysrhythmia and deliver another shock. Such delays are acceptable under ACLS standards.)

If ventricular fibrillation recurs after conversion, defibrillate again at the previously effective energy level.

To convert other dysrhythmias: Ventricular and supraventricular tachycardia require less energy for conversion. Give no more than 50 joules initially for ventricular tachycardia (unless the patient's pulseless or unresponsive). Give 25 to 100 joules for supraventricular dysrhythmias (25 joules for atrial flutter; 75 to 100 joules for paroxysmal supraventricular tachycardia or atrial fibrillation).

Synchronized cardioversion reduces the risk of triggering ventricular fibrillation. It's recommended for conversion of ventricular tachycardia (unless the patient is unconscious, pulseless, or hypotensive, or has pulmonary edema) and supraventricular rhythms.

Note: Defibrillation without a rhythm diagnosis (blind defibrillation) rarely occurs anymore, because most defibrillators in use today have monitoring ability. But ACLS standards permit blind defibrillation if no monitor's available.

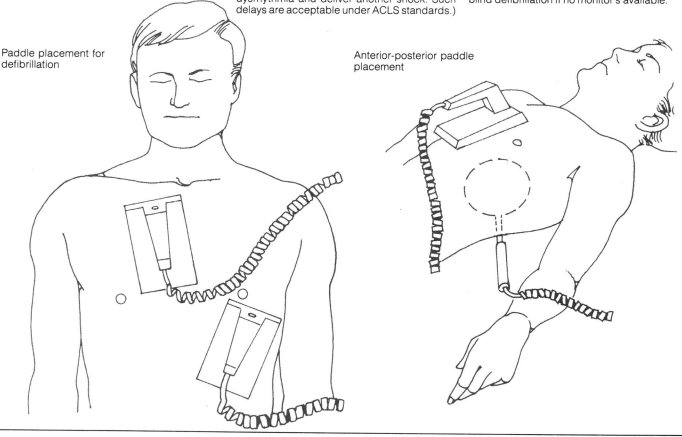

Paddle placement for defibrillation

Anterior-posterior paddle placement

Automatic external defibrillators

Research shows that a victim with ventricular fibrillation or ventricular tachycardia has a 70% chance of surviving if he's defibrillated within 3 minutes of collapse. After 20 minutes, the odds drop to 3%. Because response time for rescue squads averages about 15 minutes, an out-of-hospital victim needing defibrillation may have little chance of survival.

However, the development of automatic external defibrillators improves his odds by providing reliable defibrillator technology to emergency rescue personnel. As shown in the following photostory, an automatic defibrillator assesses heart rhythm and delivers a defibrillating shock when appropriate. Most types also have a manual mode, permitting professionals to deliver defibrillation based on their own assessment findings. Cardiac Resuscitator Corporation's versatile Heart Aid 97, the model we're featuring, can also provide automatic or manual external pacing.

These general precautions apply to any automatic defibrillator:
• Use it only if you've completed training in CPR and in operation of the device.
• Use it only if the patient's unconscious and pulseless. It's contraindicated if he's breathing.
• Don't use it on a child or small adult.
• Don't use it in a moving vehicle—movement interferes with automatic assessment.
• Don't touch the patient during the defibrillation process. (With some devices, including the Heart Aid, this includes the charging period.)
• Don't use the device near flammable gases.

Patient cable connection
Chart recorder
EKG display scope
Speaker

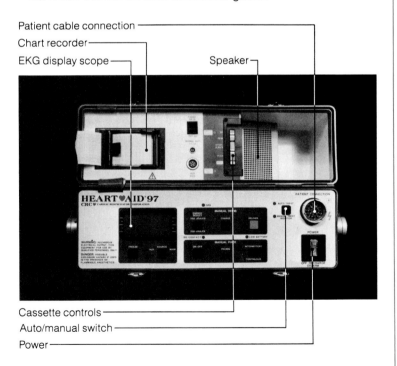

Cassette controls
Auto/manual switch
Power

Using the Heart Aid 97 automatic defibrillator

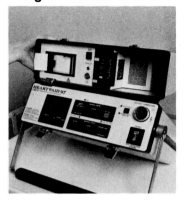

1 To prepare the Heart Aid 97 for use, remove it from its charger rack. (Battery operated, it won't function while in the charger rack.) Unlock the case, position the handle as a prop, and open the lid to reveal the upper panel (see photo).

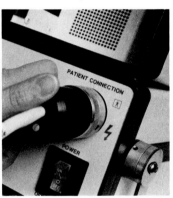

2 If the electrode cable isn't already in place, remove it from the storage pouch and attach it to the PATIENT CONNECTION outlet.

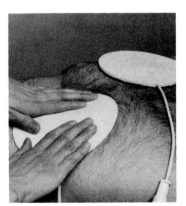

3 Remove the two electrodes from the storage pouch and remove the plastic backing. As specified by predetermined medical protocol, apply them in one of these positions: chest-chest (see photo) or chest-back. *Note:* If the preapplied electrode gel has dried or the pad looks discolored, replace the pad or moisten it with electrode gel or water.

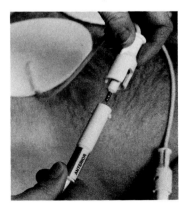

4 Connect the electrode leads to the patient cable leads. For chest-chest placement, connect the anterior (chest) electrode to the red anterior patient cable connector. Then connect the posterior (back) electrode to the white posterior cable connector.

Adult ACLS

Using the Heart Aid 97 automatic defibrillator continued

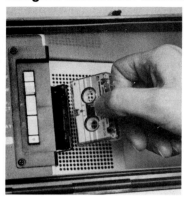

5 Insert a cassette in the tape recorder (or make sure a new tape has been installed) and latch the door shut. Depress the PLAY AND REC switches.

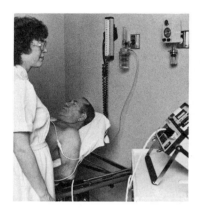

9 At this point the voice says, "STAND BACK," and you'll hear a pulsating tone. Both warnings continue for 7 to 10 seconds while charging takes place. Heart Aid continues to monitor cardiac rhythm as it charges and will abort if appropriate. Watch the display scope for the patient's EKG waveform. *Caution:* Don't touch the patient after charging begins or you may get a shock.

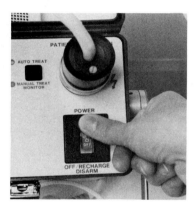

6 To initiate automatic operation, press the POWER switch on. Make sure the AUTO TREAT indicator lights up.
  Listen for the electronic voice to say, "STOP CPR." Heart Aid now automatically evaluates cardiac rhythm for at least 12 seconds.

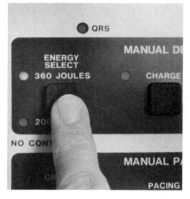

10 Count slowly to 15. If defibrillation's indicated, Heart Aid automatically delivers 200 joules within this period. (If directed by medical protocol, you can change the setting to 360 joules by pressing the ENERGY SELECT switch.) After delivering a shock, the voice says, "STAND BY," and Heart Aid resumes monitoring. A pulsating tone and the phrase "STAND BACK" indicate that Heart Aid detects VT or VF and has begun recharging.

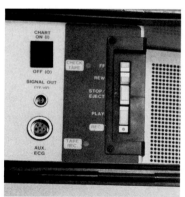

7 The TAPE REC light indicates proper tape functioning. If the CHECK TAPE indicator lights up and the voice says, "CHECK TAPE RECORDER," the tape isn't properly installed. However, Heart Aid will function normally even if you fail to correct the problem.

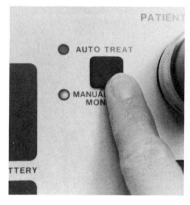

11 If the voice and tone stop, Heart Aid has aborted the shock. (You can abort defibrillation by pressing ENERGY SELECT or AUTO TREAT/ MANUAL TREAT.) If Heart Aid doesn't deliver a shock, switch to manual mode to continue monitoring. Continue the rescue protocol. *Important:* Don't resume CPR until you've switched to manual mode (or turned power off). Always use manual mode to monitor conscious patients.

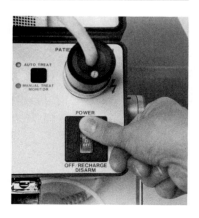

8 If you didn't place the electrodes properly, the NO CONTACT indicator lights up and the voice says, "TURN OFF HEART AID, CHECK ELECTRODES." Turn the POWER switch off and correct the problem—Heart Aid won't operate until you do. Then turn the POWER switch on, as shown.
  If Heart Aid detects ventricular tachycardia (VT) or ventricular fibrillation (VF), it begins charging for defibrillation.

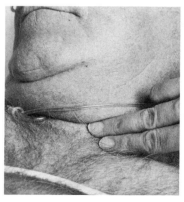

12 Heart Aid reverts to a passive monitoring cycle when it detects a heart rate between 25 and 200 beats/minute. Check the patient for pulse and breathing. If you can't detect a pulse and the equipment remains passive for 15 seconds, switch to manual mode to continue monitoring, and follow emergency protocol.

After cardiac arrest: Keeping the brain alive

Don't assume your postarrest patient has a good prognosis just because he responded to CPR within the critical 4-minute period. Brain damage can occur within even shorter periods of cerebral ischemia. What's more, the brain may continue to suffer damage after perfusion returns.

In the immediate postarrest period, cerebral ischemia causes brain dysfunction. During the reperfusion stage, more problems may arise from secondary conditions—for example, vasospasm, increased blood viscosity, hypermetabolism, and increased cellular calcium.

To preserve function, the emphasis remains on restoring cerebral perfusion as quickly as possible with basic and advanced life support. Team members should make sure that interventions intended to restore cardiac function don't jeopardize the brain. For example, they should remember that increased fluid administration to raise arterial pressure can increase intracranial pressure.

Drugs under investigation include calcium channel blockers (nimodopine and lidoflazine) to control cerebral vasospasm and improve cerebral perfusion during and after arrest, and iron-chelating agents (such as deferoxamine) to prevent cerebral degeneration postarrest.

For more brain-preserving therapies, see the chart below.

Preserving brain function with special therapies and drugs

Therapies	Purpose	Therapies	Purpose
Oxygenation	• Increases cerebral perfusion • Decreases intracranial pressure (ICP)	Hypothermia	• Reduces cerebral metabolism, decreasing the brain's need for oxygen
Hyperventilation	• Constricts cerebral vessels, reducing blood flow and lowering ICP	Hemodilution	• Decreases blood viscosity in reperfusion stage • Improves cerebral perfusion

Drugs	Purpose	Drugs	Purpose
Mannitol	• Increases cerebral perfusion • Decreases ICP	Steroids	• Decrease cerebral edema
Furosemide	• Reduces cerebral edema	Barbiturates	• Induce coma, which decreases cerebral metabolism and ICP • May also decrease ischemia

Noninvasive temporary pacemakers

Although developed 30 years ago, noninvasive temporary pacemakers have only recently come into their own as an alternative to temporary transvenous pacing. Because earlier noninvasive pacemakers caused painful stinging sensations and chest muscle contractions, few patients could tolerate them. Consequently, transvenous pacing became the preferred therapy despite its drawbacks: it requires skill and time to initiate, and it carries a high risk of such complications as pulmonary embolism, sepsis, and ventricular dysrhythmias.

Today, larger electrodes and a longer, constant-current pacing stimulus eliminate most of the discomfort associated with earlier noninvasive pacemakers. Although the anterior electrode causes chest muscle twitching, most patients don't find the sensation painful. Excessive discomfort may be relieved by slightly repositioning the electrode. (Elderly patients may experience little muscular discomfort because of age-related muscle mass losses.)

Noninvasive pacemakers require no special skill to use—just familiarity with the equipment. Unlike transvenous pacemakers, they're not associated with ventricular tachycardia or any other complication. In addition to emergency use, they can be used prophylactically during permanent pacemaker insertion.

Read the following photostory for how to use the Zoll NTP (noninvasive temporary pacemaker). Consult the manufacturer's instructions for more details.

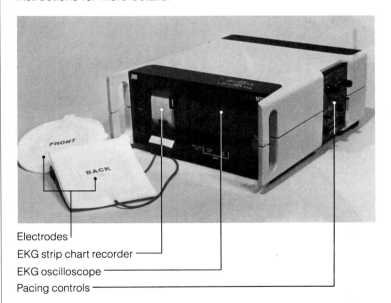

Electrodes
EKG strip chart recorder
EKG oscilloscope
Pacing controls

Adult ACLS

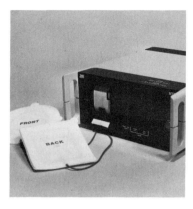

1 Weighing only 18 lb, the Zoll NTP (noninvasive temporary pacemaker) operates as a demand pacemaker in the VVI mode. It runs on wall or battery power and can be used for adults and children.

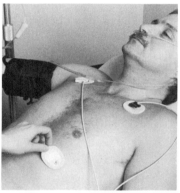

2 Connect the patient to the cardiac monitor, and make sure you have a good EKG tracing. If the patient's conscious, explain the procedure and answer his questions. Tell him he'll feel chest muscle twitching during pacing but that it shouldn't be painful. *Important:* Don't neglect to prepare the patient. Anxiety decreases his ability to tolerate the procedure.

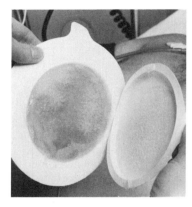

3 Using the tab, peel the protective cap from the BACK electrode. Don't let the electrode gel contaminate the adhesive border, or the electrode won't adhere properly.

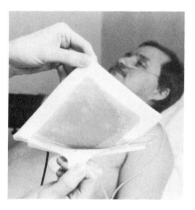

4 Dry the skin (if time permits) and place the electrode between the left scapula and spine at midheart level. (Avoid damaged skin, if possible.) Press the adhesive border (rather than the electrode's center portion) against the skin.

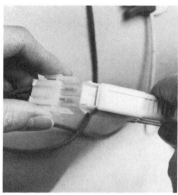

5 Peel off the FRONT electrode cover and apply the electrode in the V_3–V_4 area on a male patient. (Don't shave the area.) For a female patient, apply it under the left breast.

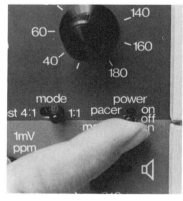

6 Connect the electrodes to the output cable. (Always apply the electrodes to the patient before connecting them to the cable.)

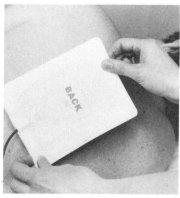

7 Set the power switch to PACER ON, as shown here. Set the pacing rate at a value above the patient's heart rate. Then, starting from zero, increase the pacing output current until you see evidence of capture. Set the output at 10% above the minimum level for effective stimulation. (For most patients, this falls between 40 and 80 milliamperes.) *Caution:* Don't touch an electrode's gelled side after turning on the power.

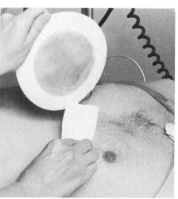

8 Before removing a pacer electrode, first set the power switch to OFF or MONITOR. Then wipe off any excess gel on the skin—gel can form an electrical pathway between electrodes.

Pediatric ACLS

Most pediatric cardiac arrests stem from a respiratory problem, such as near drowning, not a primary dysrhythmia. The victims—most of them younger than age 1—include sudden infant death syndrome infants. Even with CPR, mortality exceeds 90%.

As with adult advanced cardiac life support (ACLS), pediatric ACLS begins with basic life support, which we discussed beginning on page 6. In the following pages, we'll cover current standards for drug and adjunctive equipment use during a pediatric emergency.

Selecting an endotracheal tube

Use this chart as a guide only. If a child's large or small for his age, he may need a tube that's one size larger or smaller than indicated here.

Age	Internal diameter (mm)
Newborn	3.0
6 mo	3.5
18 mo	4.0
3 yr	4.5
5 yr	5.0
6 yr	5.5
8 yr	6.0
12 yr	6.5
16 yr	7.0
Adult (F)	7.5-8.0
Adult (M)	8.0-8.5

Intubating a child: Points to remember

A child's airway becomes narrowest at the cricoid cartilage (rather than at the glottic opening, where an adult's airway narrows). Consequently, the doctor may have difficulty advancing an endotracheal (ET) tube at the cricoid level. Other differences from adult anatomy include a more flexible and proportionately smaller airway, a proportionately larger tongue, and a glottic opening located higher in the neck. Using appropriate equipment and techniques minimizes insertion problems.

Indications for ET tube insertion include inability to ventilate an unconscious patient, cardiac or respiratory arrest, and a need for prolonged artificial ventilation. Follow these guidelines:
• Choose a tube appropriate for the child's size (see the chart at left).
• Use an uncuffed tube for a child younger than age 8; a cuffed tube for older children.
• Obtain a stylet or a straight or curved laryngoscope blade to help provide rigidity and guide the tube through the child's vocal cords. (The doctor will probably prefer a straight blade for an infant.)
• Give artificial ventilation, preferably with supplemental oxygen, before insertion.
• During insertion, constantly monitor heart rate. If it falls below 60 beats/minute (below 80 beats/minute for an infant), stop the procedure and provide artificial ventilation. *Important:* Don't allow more than 30 seconds to pass without ventilating the patient.

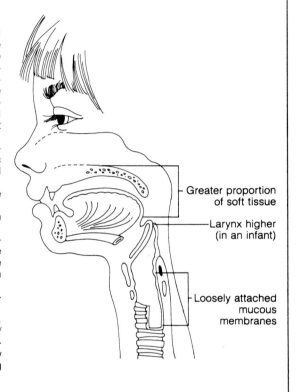

Greater proportion of soft tissue

Larynx higher (in an infant)

Loosely attached mucous membranes

Defibrillation and cardioversion update

If you find a child unconscious and pulseless, immediately begin CPR to restore ventilation, oxygenation, and circulation. Prepare to defibrillate only if EKG monitoring identifies ventricular fibrillation. Don't perform blind defibrillation (defibrillation without a rhythm diagnosis) on an infant or a child.

Choose the largest chest electrodes that adhere evenly to the child's chest. In general, use paddles 4.5 cm in diameter for infants and 8 cm in diameter for older children.

Current standards recommend an initial shock of 2 joules/kg. If this fails to defibrillate, double the energy dose and repeat twice. If three shocks fail to convert the dysrhythmia, take action to correct acidosis, hypoxemia, and hypothermia, as necessary. Continue basic life-support procedures and give epinephrine (and

possibly lidocaine) to facilitate defibrillation, as ordered.

After successfully converting ventricular fibrillation, the doctor may order bretylium or lidocaine to raise the fibrillation threshold. If fibrillation recurs, current standards recommend that you *don't* raise the energy level for defibrillation above the previously successful level.

Indications for synchronized cardioversion include symptomatic supraventricular or ventricular tachycardias. Give one tenth to one half the defibrillation energy dose (0.2 to 1 joule/kg). Begin at a low dose and gradually increase the dose if necessary. Correct acidosis, hypoxemia, hypoglycemia, and hypothermia, as needed.

Pediatric ACLS

Emergency drugs: Pediatric guidelines

Bradycardia and asystole, the commonest pediatric dysrhythmias, respond best to epinephrine. Because acidosis depresses the action of epinephrine and other catecholamines, maintaining ventilation and circulation during therapy becomes crucial. *Important:* Don't administer catecholamines in the same I.V. line as an alkaline solution, such as sodium bicarbonate. Alkalis inactivate catecholamines.

Fewer than 10% of pediatric cardiac arrests involve ventricular fibrillation or ventricular tachycardia. When present, such dysrhythmias may reflect an electrolyte imbalance, abnormal glucose levels, hypothermia, or drug-related problems. Ventricular dysrhythmias respond best to lidocaine.

Consult the chart at right for information on pediatric ACLS drugs. When possible, administer drugs directly into the central circulation; make peripheral venous insertion your second choice. In larger children, drug administration at a supradiaphragmatic site provides faster access to the central circulation than does administration below the diaphragm; in smaller children, however, this consideration seems less important.

Establishing venous access may be difficult in a child, particularly during an emergency. As an alternative, the doctor may choose the intraosseous route. Using a rigid needle (such as a bone marrow needle or a spinal needle with a stylet), he can inject drugs into the anterior tibial bone marrow, a noncollapsible venous plexus that rapidly absorbs catecholamines and bicarbonate.

In the absence of venous or intraosseous access, you can give epinephrine, atropine, and lidocaine endotracheally. Give no less than the dose you'd give I.V. To enhance delivery, dilute the drug into 1 to 2 ml of normal saline solution.

Consider intracardiac injection the route of last resort.

Pediatric ACLS drugs

The following chart provides details on front-line pediatric ACLS drugs. Dosages apply to I.V. or endotracheal administration. For details on preparing I.V. infusions, see the guidelines on the opposite page.

Atropine sulfate

Indications
• Symptomatic bradycardia (or heart rate below 80 beats/minute in a distressed infant younger than age 6 months, with or without hypotension)
• Vagally mediated bradycardia during endotracheal intubation
• Ventricular asystole
• Symptomatic bradycardia with atrioventricular block (rare)

Dosage
0.02 mg/kg/dose. If necessary, repeat in 5 minutes. Maximum total dosage: 1 mg for children; 2 mg for adolescents.

Pediatric considerations
• Give no less than 0.1 mg. Smaller doses may trigger paradoxical bradycardia.
• Monitor the patient for tachycardia, a common side effect.
• If giving atropine to block bradycardia during intubation, keep in mind that atropine may mask hypoxemia-induced bradycardia. Minimize risk of hypoxemia by avoiding prolonged intubation attempts.

Calcium chloride

Indications
• Hypocalcemia
• Hyperkalemia
• Hypermagnesemia
• Calcium channel blocker overdose. *Important:* Calcium *not* recommended during resuscitation efforts unless hypocalcemia is clearly present.

Dosage
20 mg/kg/dose. Repeat in 10 minutes, if necessary.

Pediatric considerations
• Infuse slowly.
• Base subsequent dosage on documented calcium deficits.

Dobutamine hydrochloride

Indications
• Poor myocardial function from diminished cardiac output

Dosage
5 to 15 mcg/kg/min

Pediatric considerations
• Monitor dosage closely. Overdose may cause tachycardia or ventricular ectopy.
• The doctor may order dobutamine for a patient who fails to respond to dopamine.

Dopamine hydrochloride

Indications
• Shock
• Hypotension or poor peripheral perfusion postresuscitation

Dosage
5 to 10 mcg/kg/min initially; increase to a maximum of 20 mcg/kg/min if necessary to improve blood pressure, perfusion, and urine output

Pediatric considerations
• Dosage determines dopamine's effects. At a dosage above 20 mcg/kg/min, dopamine may cause excessive vasoconstriction and its renal vasodilating effect diminishes.
• After reaching the maximum dosage, the doctor may order epinephrine or dobutamine for further inotropic effects.
• Tape I.V. device securely and monitor for infiltration, which could cause a chemical burn.
• Monitor for adverse effects: tachycardia, severe vasoconstriction, ventricular ectopy.

Epinephrine hydrochloride

Indications
• Asystole
• Bradydysrhythmias

Dosage
0.01 mg/kg (0.1 ml/kg of 1:10,000 solution). Repeat every 5 minutes, as needed.

Pediatric considerations
• At high doses, epinephrine can cause excessive vasoconstriction, compromising blood flow to extremities and internal organs (particularly the kidneys).

• The doctor may order epinephrine as a continuous I.V. infusion (preferably into a central vein) to treat hypotension or poor perfusion postresuscitation or to treat symptomatic bradycardia unresponsive to atropine.
• Monitor I.V. insertion site for infiltration.

Isoproterenol hydrochloride

Indications
• Hemodynamically significant bradycardia resistant to atropine
• Heart block (rare in children)

Dosage
0.1 to 1 mcg/kg/min

Pediatric considerations
• Monitor the patient for tachycardia.

Lidocaine hydrochloride

Indications
• Ventricular fibrillation
• Ventricular tachycardia
• Ventricular ectopy causing hypotension and poor perfusion

Dosage
1 mg/kg/dose initially as a bolus

Pediatric considerations
• Give lidocaine before electrical therapy (cardioversion or defibrillation), if possible; however, don't delay electrical therapy if drug isn't available.
• Begin an I.V. infusion (20 to 50 mcg/kg/min) if electrical therapy and a bolus dose don't correct ventricular tachycardia or ventricular fibrillation. To ensure adequate blood levels, give another bolus dose before beginning the infusion.

• Reduce the infusion rate in shock, congestive heart failure, and cardiac arrest: drug clearance slows under these circumstances. Monitor the patient for myocardial and circulatory depression and for central nervous system effects (drowsiness, muscle twitching, disorientation, seizures). Discontinue the infusion if such adverse effects develop.

Sodium bicarbonate

Indications
• Prolonged cardiac arrest or unstable hemodynamic state with documented metabolic acidosis. *Note:* Sodium bicarbonate is not normally indicated during resuscitation efforts.

Dosage
1 mEq/kg (1 ml/kg of 8.4% solution) in children; for infants, dilute to 0.5 mEq/ml

Pediatric considerations
• If possible, base subsequent doses on acid-base measurements. If not available, the doctor may give doses at 10-minute intervals during a prolonged arrest.

Pediatric dosages at a glance
This chart provides dosages for several pediatric ACLS drugs, based on a child's weight. Under each drug name, you'll find first the drug concentration, then the standard pediatric dose. *Important:* Never change the concentration.

To estimate your patient's weight, use this formula:
weight in kg = 8 + (age × 2).

WEIGHT IN KG	5	10	15	20	25	30	35	40	45	50
EPINEPHRINE 1:10,000 0.1 mg/ml— 0.01 mg/kg	0.5 ml	1 ml	1.5 ml	2 ml	2.5 ml	3 ml	3.5 ml	4 ml	4.5 ml	5 ml
SODIUM BICARBONATE 1 mEq/ml— 1 ml/kg	5 ml	10 ml	15 ml	20 ml	25 ml	30 ml	35 ml	40 ml	45 ml	50 ml
ATROPINE 0.1 mg/ml— 0.01 mg/kg	1.5 ml	1.5 ml	1.5 ml	2 ml	2.5 ml	3 ml	3.5 ml	4 ml	4.5 ml	5 ml
CALCIUM CHLORIDE 100 mg/ml— 10 mg/kg 10%	0.5 ml	1 ml	1.5 ml	2 ml	2.5 ml	3 ml	3.5 ml	4 ml	4.5 ml	5 ml
LIDOCAINE 20 mg/ml— 1 mg/kg	0.25 ml	0.5 ml	0.75 ml	1 ml	1.25 ml	1.5 ml	1.75 ml	2 ml	2.25 ml	2.5 ml

SPECIAL CONSIDERATIONS

Preparing a pediatric I.V. infusion

Epinephrine, isoproterenol, norepinephrine
To prepare:
Multiply 0.6 × body weight (in kg) for drug dose (in mg). Add drug to diluent (dextrose 5% in water [D₅W], dextrose 5% in half normal saline solution, normal saline solution, or Ringer's lactate) to make 100 ml.
Dosage:
1 ml/hr delivers 0.1 /mcg/kg/min; titrate to effect.

Dobutamine, dopamine
To prepare:
Multiply 6 × body weight (in kg) for drug dose (in mg). Add drug to diluent (D₅W, dextrose 5% in half normal saline solution, normal saline solution, or Ringer's lactate) to make 100 ml.
Dosage:
1 ml/hr delivers 1 mcg/kg/min; titrate to effect.

Lidocaine
To prepare:
Add 120 mg (3 ml of 4% solution) to 100 ml of D₅W to make 1,200 mcg/ml.
Dosage:
1 ml/kg/hr delivers 20 mcg/kg/min.

Neonatal ACLS

Every year, about 3.5 million babies are born in 5,000 United States hospitals. Approximately 6% of these new-borns require life support in the delivery room; among babies weighing less than 1,500 g, 80% need life support. Yet only 15% of hospitals with delivery facilities have neonatal intensive care units.

The American Heart Association urges hospitals to develop in-house programs to teach neonatal resuscitation standards and skills. The next few pages highlight current recommendations.

SPECIAL CONSIDERATIONS

Neonatal resuscitation guidelines

The Apgar neonatal assessment system shown at right indicates a newborn infant's overall health by assigning him a score based on his heart rate, respirations, muscle tone, reflex irritability, and color. Normally, Apgar scoring reflects the infant's status 1 minute and 5 minutes after his complete birth (with reassessment every 5 minutes following a 5-minute score below 7). If indicated, however, begin resuscitation efforts immediately without waiting for even a 1-minute score.

Heart rate, respiration, and color provide the best indicators of neonatal distress. Assess heart rate by listening to the apical heartbeat with a stethoscope, feeling the pulse at the umbilical cord's base, or monitoring with a cardiotachometer.

Administer neonatal resuscitation in four steps:
- Position, suction, and stimulate.
- Ventilate with bag, mask, and endotracheal tube (if necessary).
- Perform chest compressions.
- Give drugs and fluids.

Most infants respond to the first two steps; only a few need chest compressions and drugs. Nevertheless, every delivery room team should be prepared to handle a crisis. At least one person who's skilled at neonatal resuscitation should be present at every delivery. Another skilled professional should be readily available, because life support for a severely depressed and asphyxiated infant requires intubation and closely coordinated ventilations and chest compressions. During prolonged resuscitation efforts, a third person should be ready to insert I.V. catheters and administer drugs.

Read the following pages for details on resuscitation measures. *Important:* Hypothermia, a particular danger to asphyxiated infants, delays recovery from acidosis. Prevent heat loss by keeping the delivery room warm, placing the infant under a warmer immediately after birth, and drying him quickly.

Understanding the Apgar scoring system

Reliable and widely accepted, the Apgar scoring system allows you to establish baseline assessment findings quickly.

Rate each of the following five indicators on a scale from 0 (very poor) to 2 (excellent). Add the points to obtain the infant's total score. An infant scoring below 6 may require resuscitation.

Remember these points during your assessment:
- *Heart rate.* This indicator is the most important—and the last to be absent if an infant's in distress. Within the first few minutes of birth, a normal infant's heart rate is between 150 and 180 beats/minute; it then decreases to between 130 and 140 beats/minute. A rate below 100 beats/minute suggests asphyxia.

For the most accurate assessment, determine apical heart rate with a pediatric stethoscope. You can also determine heart rate by palpating the umbilical cord.
- *Respiratory effort:* Within 2 minutes after birth, an infant should breathe spontaneously and regularly at a rate of 35 to 50 breaths/minute.
- *Muscle tone:* A normal infant keeps his arms and legs flexed and resists your efforts to straighten them.
- *Reflex irritability.* Normally, an infant coughs, sneezes, and cries during suctioning; he also protests against tactile stimulation (for example, flicking the soles of his feet).
- *Skin color.* An infant appears cyanotic at birth, but his trunk acquires normal coloring within 3 minutes. (His arms and legs may remain blue longer.)

Indicator	0	1	2
Heart rate	Absent	Less than 100 beats/minute	More than 100 beats/minute
Respiratory effort	Absent	Slow, irregular, weak cry	Good, vigorous cry
Muscle tone	Flaccid, limp	Some flexion of extremities	Good flexion, active motion
Reflex irritability (in response to catheter in nostril)	No response	Weak cry or grimace	Vigorous cry, cough, sneeze
Skin color	Blue	Body skin color normal (depending on infant's race), extremities blue	Body and extremity skin color normal

Step 1: Positioning, suctioning, and stimulation

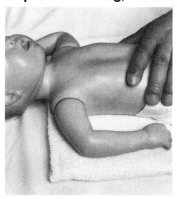

1 For demonstration purposes, we're using a Resusci-Baby in this photostory.
Position the infant on his back or left side in a slight Trendelenburg position, with his neck in a neutral position. (Overextension or underextension may obstruct his airway.) Place a 1″ thick blanket or towel under his shoulders to help maintain head position.

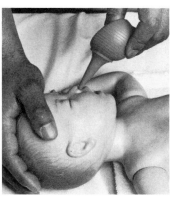

2 Suction with a bulb syringe, DeLee trap, or mechanical suction device attached to a suction catheter (see chart at right for sizes). Avoid pressures exceeding −100 mm Hg (−136 cm of water). Limit suctioning to less than 10 seconds at a time, and monitor for bradycardia and apnea (possible consequences of deep suctioning, which may produce a vagal response).

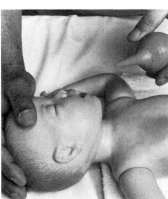

3 Between suctionings, give the infant time to breathe spontaneously, or provide ventilatory assistance with 100% oxygen. (To guard against meconium aspiration, the doctor suctions as soon as the infant's head is delivered, if possible.)

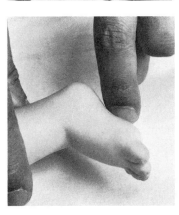

4 If suctioning doesn't stimulate effective respirations, try slapping or flicking the soles of the infant's feet, or rub his back. Avoid more vigorous methods.

Step 2: Ventilation

Most infants needing ventilatory support respond to assistance from positive-pressure ventilation. Initial lung inflation may require pressure between 30 and 40 cm of water; subsequent inflations should require less pressure. While providing a ventilatory rate of 40 breaths/minute, watch for bilateral lung expansion and auscultate for breath sounds. Also watch for a distended stomach, which may require periodic decompression.

If you can't inflate the lungs adequately, first suction, then reposition the head and face mask. If the problem persists, the doctor will perform a laryngoscopic examination of the upper airway and intubate the trachea. Other indications for intubation include apnea, a heart rate below 100 beats/minute, and persistent central cyanosis despite administration of 100% oxygen.

After you've established adequate ventilation for 15 to 30 seconds, your next step depends on the heart rate. Follow these guidelines:
• *Heart rate greater than 100 beats/minute; spontaneous respiration:* Discontinue positive-pressure ventilation. Maintain spontaneous respiration with gentle tactile stimulation. If spontaneous respiration ceases, resume positive-pressure ventilation.
• *Heart rate below 60 beats/minute:* Continue positive-pressure ventilation and begin chest compressions.
• *Heart rate 60 to 100 beats/minute and rising:* Continue assisted ventilation; discontinue chest compressions.
• *Heart rate 60 to 100 beats/minute and not rising:* Make sure you're providing adequate ventilation. If the heart rate remains below 80 beats/minute, begin chest compressions.

Tube and catheter sizes

Infant weight, g	Endotracheal tube diameter, mm (inside)	Suction catheter size
<1,000	2.5	5F
1,000 to 2,000	3.0	6F
2,000 to 3,000	3.5	8F
>3,000	4.0	8F

Neonatal ACLS

Step 3: Chest compressions

To perform chest compressions on an infant, position your fingers in one of the ways shown on the Resusci-Baby featured below. Compress the sternum ½" to ¾" at a rate of 120 compressions/minute in smooth, even motions. Make sure compression time equals relaxation time, and take care not to lift your fingers from the sternum during relaxation.

Provide positive-pressure ventilation with 100% oxygen at a rate of 40 to 60 breaths/minute. (Current standards don't provide recommendations on how to coordinate ventilations and chest compressions.)

Check the pulse rate regularly and discontinue chest compressions when the heart rate reaches 80 beats/minute or more. Note: Recent research establishes that an infant's heart lies lower (in relation to external landmarks) than previously thought. Thus, current standards recommend a lower compression area.

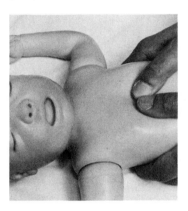

1 For a small infant, use the technique shown here. With your fingers supporting the back, place your two thumbs on the sternum's middle third just below an imaginary line between the nipples. *Caution:* Don't compress the sternum's lower portion—you could damage internal organs.

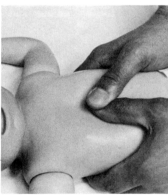

2 On a very small infant, your thumbs may overlap, as in this photo.

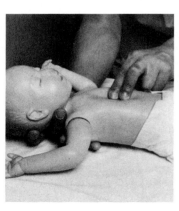

3 For a larger infant, use the two-finger compression method shown here. Place two fingers on the sternum one finger's width below the nipple line. You can use your other hand to support the infant's back and maintain the head tilt.

Step 4: Drugs and fluids

During neonatal resuscitation efforts, the umbilical vein provides the preferred administration route. (An umbilical artery may also be used, but it's more difficult to cannulate.) Obtain a 3.5F or 5F umbilical catheter with a radiopaque marker. The doctor advances it until its tip rests just below skin level. Peripheral or scalp veins, while also an option, may be difficult to cannulate in an emergency.

To administer epinephrine when the I.V. route isn't available, use the endotracheal route. As with adults, use the same dosage recommended for the I.V. route (see the following information). Dilute epinephrine (1:10,000) with 1 to 2 ml of normal saline solution to aid drug delivery.

Recommendations for drug and fluid administration

Current standards don't recommend calcium or atropine during the acute phase of neonatal resuscitation. Similarly, sodium bicarbonate shouldn't be given routinely; oxygenation and ventilation provide the best weapons against hypoxemia and acidosis. Without them, sodium bicarbonate won't improve blood pH.

Drugs and fluids appropriate during resuscitation include:
• *epinephrine hydrochloride.* In addition to improving perfusion pressure through vasodilation, epinephrine enhances myocardial contractility and raises the heart rate. It's indicated in asystole and when the spontaneous heart rate falls below 80 beats/minute despite ventilation with 100% oxygen and chest compressions. As ordered, give 0.01 to 0.03 mg/kg (0.1 to 0.3 ml/kg of the 1:10,000 solution) I.V or endotracheally. Repeat every 5 minutes, if needed.
• *volume expanders.* These fluids correct hypovolemia, a likely complication in any infant needing resuscitation. Indications include acute bleeding from the infant/maternal unit, persistent pallor despite oxygenation, faint pulses despite a good heart rate, and poor response to assisted ventilation and other resuscitation efforts. The doctor may order:
—10 ml/kg of O-negative blood cross-matched with the mother's blood
—10 ml/kg of 5% albumin/saline solution (or another plasma substitute)
—10 ml/kg of normal saline solution or Ringer's lactate.
Note: Give volume expanders over 5 to 10 minutes.
• *naloxone hydrochloride.* If the mother received narcotics within 4 hours of delivery (or if she's a narcotics addict), the neonate may need naloxone to reverse narcotic-induced respiratory depression. Precede drug administration with ventilatory assistance. *Important:* Use naloxone cautiously if the mother's an addict—the drug may trigger withdrawal symptoms in the infant.

Give 0.01 mg/kg of a neonatal solution (Narcan Neonatal, 0.02 mg/ml) I.V., endotracheally, or (with adequate perfusion) subcutaneously or intramuscularly. Monitor the infant closely for a return of respiratory depression—the narcotic's effects may outlast naloxone's countereffects. Repeat the initial dose every 2 minutes, as necessary.

Shock and trauma care

If you've ever cared for a patient who's in shock or who has traumatic injuries, you know that his recovery may depend on your up-to-date knowledge of the latest medical procedures and equipment. On the next few pages, we familiarize you with a few special procedures and devices that can improve your patient's survival odds and reduce the risk of serious complications. You'll learn how to:
• use the trauma score to assess an accident victim
• set up and use autotransfusion equipment
• perform ocular lavage using the Morgan Therapeutic Lens.

We'll also acquaint you with the Infuser37, a rapid blood-infusion device that replaces lost blood and fluids quickly, with little risk of transfusion hypothermia.

Read what follows for details.

UPDATE

Trauma care: Current assessment guidelines

You're working in the emergency department when a rescue squad brings in 29-year-old Jim Jacobs. You learn that Mr. Jacobs has suffered multiple trauma from a motorcycle accident. To give him the best chance of survival, you must perform a fast, accurate nursing assessment based on his trauma score and the accident history.

Developed to aid assessment shortly after a traumatic injury, the trauma score (see page 30) incorporates both cardiopulmonary findings (blood pressure, capillary refill, respiratory rate, and respiratory effort) with neurologic findings reflected by the Glasgow Coma Scale. Your patient's score indicates the severity of injuries and predicts his survival chances.

Take a look at the projected survival estimates in the box on page 30. As you see, the higher the score, the better the patient's chances. Trauma scores become critically important when you have several trauma patients to assess, because they help you determine who needs treatment first and who needs transfer to a trauma center.

Determining trauma score
To assign Mr. Jacobs a trauma score, follow these steps:
• Count his respiratory rate and assign the appropriate point value. Mr. Jacobs' respiratory rate is 40, so assign 2 points.
• Assess respiratory effort. In Mr. Jacobs' case it's labored, so you assign 0 points.
• Check his blood pressure. Because his systolic pressure is 69 mm Hg palpable, you assign 2 points.

• Test capillary refill by blanching a fingernail bed and counting the seconds until blood returns. Refill takes longer than 2 seconds, so assign 1 point.
• Determine neurologic status with the Glasgow Coma Scale. Your findings: the patient opens his eyes only when you call his name (3 points), he seems confused when you ask him the date (4 points), and he shows purposeful movement by pushing your hand away when you attempt to elicit a pain response (5 points). Adding these points gives you a Glasgow Coma Scale score of 12, which counts as 4 points toward the total trauma score. (The key titled *GCS score* near the bottom of the trauma score scale indicates how to weigh points.)

The patient's points total 9, a score associated with a 37% survival rate. You draw two conclusions: he has serious injuries, and he may require transfer to a trauma center. *Remember:* Use discretion when you report your findings. Don't allow the patient or his family to overhear bad news.

Assessing mechanism of injury
Your assessment isn't complete until you learn as much as possible about the accident. For example, what caused the accident? How fast was the patient driving at the time? Was he wearing a seatbelt? All this information helps the doctor evaluate the nature of the injury and begin appropriate treatment. The box below indicates how all your findings contribute to triage.

Continue to reassess the patient frequently—his condition could deteriorate suddenly.

MINI-ASSESSMENT

Guidelines for transfer to a trauma center

A patient who meets any of these criteria probably needs care at a trauma center.

Physical assessment
• Trauma score below 12
• Glasgow Coma Scale score below 10
• Systolic blood pressure below 90 mm Hg
• Respiratory rate below 10
• Spinal cord injury
• Two or more proximal long-bone fractures
• Penetrating injury to head, neck, abdomen, chest, or groin
• Injuries involving two or more body systems
• Burns in the airway or on the face
• Burns covering 15% or more of body surface area
• Paralysis
• Amputation above the ankle or wrist

• Flail chest
• Age less than 5 or more than 55 years
• History of cardiac or respiratory disease

Mechanism of injury
• Fall from 15'
• Accident involving a hostile environment (for example, water or temperature extremes)
• Car crash at a speed above 20 mph
• Passenger compartment intrusion of 18"
• Death of another passenger in car
• Victim ejected from car
• Victim trapped in car for 20 minutes
• Victim struck by car moving at 20 mph

Shock and trauma care

Trauma score

A. Respiratory rate	10-24/min	4
	25-35/min	3
	36/min or greater	2
	1-9/min	1
	None	0
B. Respiratory effort	Normal	1
	Shallow or retractive	0
C. Systolic blood pressure	90 mm Hg or greater	4
	70-89 mm Hg	3
	50-69 mm Hg	2
	0-49 mm Hg	1
	No pulse	0
D. Capillary refill	Normal (within 2 seconds)	2
	Delayed (> 2 seconds)	1
	None	0

E. Glasgow Coma Scale (GCS)
  1. Eye opening
Spontaneous	4
To voice	3
To pain	2
None	1

  2. Verbal response
Oriented	5
Confused	4
Inappropriate words	3
Incomprehensible words	2
None	1

  3. Motor response
Obeys command	6
Localizes pain	5
Withdrawn (pain)	4
Flexion (pain)	3
Extension (pain)	2
None	1

Total GCS points: _____

GCS score:
14-15 = 5
11-13 = 4
 8-10 = 3
 5-7 = 2
 3-4 = 1

Total trauma score
(add trauma points [A+B+C+D]
and GCS score): _____

Survival estimates

About 90% of all trauma victims score 13 or better on the trauma score scale.

Trauma score		Percentage who survive
16	90% of patients	99
15		98
14		95
13		91
12	10% of patients	83
11		71
10		55
9		37
8		22
7		12
6		7
5		4
4		2
3		1
2		0
1		0

Warming crystalloid solutions by microwave

As you know, administering room-temperature I.V. solutions to a hypovolemic patient can trigger hypothermia. Yet he may need fluids so urgently that you haven't time to warm them by conventional methods.

An ordinary microwave oven can solve this dilemma for you. In it, you can rapidly warm Ringer's lactate or normal saline solution for infusion. (Warm only nondextrose crystalloid solutions by microwave.) Follow this procedure:
• Place a 1,000-ml bag of the ordered solution into a 650-watt microwave oven (without turntable).
• Close the oven door and turn on the high setting for 1 minute.
• After 1 minute, remove the bag, agitate it for 2 or 3 seconds, and replace it in the oven face-down.
• Again turn on the high setting for 1 minute.
• If time permits, test solution temperature by placing a digital thermometer probe between folded ends of the solution bag.
• Agitate the heated solution before spiking and hanging the bag for infusion.

Using the Bard Infuser37 for rapid fluid administration

For a patient with multiple injuries, bleeding can quickly lead to life-threatening hypovolemia. Along with stopping the bleeding, replacing lost fluid becomes a top priority. When you need to restore fluid volume rapidly, the Bard Infuser37 featured here can be a lifesaver.

How it works

A rapid solution infusion system, the Bard Infuser37 can provide the patient with blood and crystalloids at high flow rates: packed cells and whole blood at rates of 700 ml/minute or more; crystalloids at 1,800 ml/minute. Its built-in heat exchanger, easily attached to a water heater, warms the fluids to 98.6° F. (37° C.) to reduce the risk of transfusion-induced hypothermia.

As shown at right, the system consists of a Y-shaped infusion line with two input branches: a 40-micron filtered branch for the primary blood infusion and an unfiltered branch for fluid infusion. (If the patient needs multiple blood transfusions, you can add a filter to this branch and use it for transfusion.) As you see, the system also has two injection ports and a secondary line you can attach to administer medication or to maintain a keep-vein-open infusion rate. Safety features include a ball valve that prevents air embolism if an I.V. container empties and a 170-micron screen filter near the patient.

Precautions

Before using the Infuser37, consult product inserts for indications, contraindications, directions for use, warnings, and precautions. Here are a few important points:
• Don't use the Infuser37 unless you've completed hands-on training.
• It's contraindicated for a patient with a condition (such as a septal defect) that allows venous and arterial blood to mix. Use it with caution if the patient has congestive heart failure, obstructive uropathy, or renal insufficiency.
• Prime the system with fluid before attaching it to the patient.
• For maximum flow rates, use an 8.5F (or larger) venous catheter.
• Don't let water inlet pressure within the heat exchanger exceed 65 psi; don't let temperature exceed 107.6° F. (42° C.).
• If you use a pressure cuff on the blood bag, don't let pressure exceed 300 mm Hg.
• To avoid potential hypervolemia from fluid overload, monitor the patient closely throughout therapy.
• Replace the system every 24 hours; replace the blood filters more frequently, as needed. Don't sterilize and reuse the system.

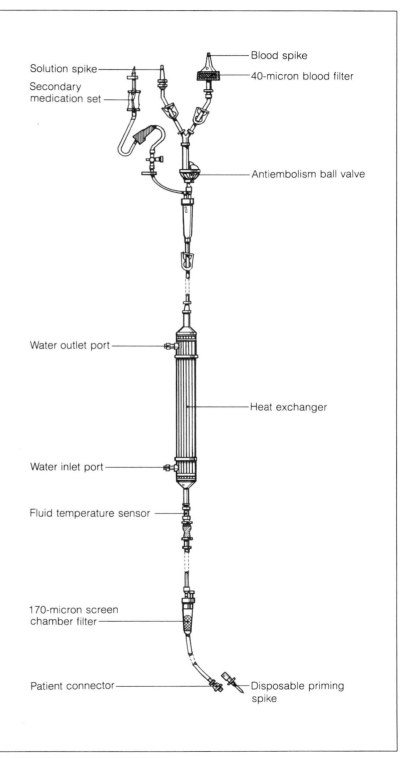

Shock and trauma care

Autotransfusion: A growing role in emergency care

Thanks to safer, simpler equipment and techniques, autotransfusion—the collection, filtration, and reinfusion of a patient's own blood—has become a widely accepted procedure in emergency departments and trauma centers. Used mostly for patients with chest wounds, it's indicated whenever 2 or 3 units of pooled blood can be recovered from a wound or body cavity.

Autotransfusion also plays an important part in emergency and nonemergency surgery. Blood may be obtained:
• *preoperatively.* A patient can donate his blood for storage and later use during elective surgery up to 35 days in advance. He can donate as often as every 5 days up to 5 days before surgery. Even patients with conditions that normally rule out blood donation can donate for autotransfusion.
• *immediately before surgery.* After anesthetizing the patient, the doctor can withdraw 1 to 2 units of blood and replace the volume with crystalloid or colloid solution to provide fresh, warm, compatible blood for immediate use. (This procedure is most common in cardiovascular and orthopedic procedures.)
• *during surgery.* The doctor can collect shed blood from a wound or body cavity, then reinfuse it.
• *postoperatively.* Blood shed during surgery can be collected and replaced in the recovery room or surgical intensive care unit.

Pros and cons

The doctor may order autotransfusion instead of a stored blood transfusion because autotransfusion:
• eliminates the risk of transfusion reactions and transmission of such diseases as hepatitis, malaria, and acquired immune deficiency syndrome
• provides compatible blood immediately by eliminating the usual 45-minute period required for blood typing and cross matching
• reduces transfusion costs (blood for autotransfusion is up to six times cheaper per unit than donor blood)
• prevents transfusion hypothermia because the blood's already warm
• avoids hypokalemia, hypocalcemia, and acidosis because the blood has normal levels of potassium, ammonia, hydrogen ions, and 2,3-diphosphoglycerate, which helps oxygenate tissues
• reduces the risk of overtransfusion and subsequent circulatory overload
• conserves stored blood supplies
• may be given to patients with rare blood types and those with religious objections to homologous blood transfusions.

Possible complications of autotransfusion include hematologic changes (such as decreased platelet and fibrinogen levels and abnormal platelet function), coagulopathy, sepsis, microembolism, and air embolism. However, a recent study found that only 4% of 300 high-risk patients experienced adverse reactions to autotransfusion, and none developed a serious problem. (To learn how to reduce the risk of adverse effects, see page 37.)

On the following pages, you'll learn how to operate two widely used autotransfusion devices—the Pleur-evac ATS, made by the Deknatel Division of Pfizer Hospital Products Group, Inc., and the Receptal ATS, made by Sorenson Research Co. Easy to use, both systems reduce the risk of error during an emergency. They also contain special equipment that minimizes blood cell damage during collection, reduces the risk of air embolism during transfusion, and filters out microaggregates.

Performing autotransfusion with the Pleur-evac ATS

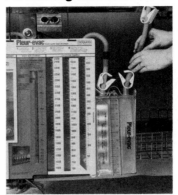

1 First, establish underwater seal drainage and connect the patient's chest tube by following steps 1 through 4 printed on the front of the Pleur-evac unit. Inspect the blood collection bag and tubing, making sure all clamps are open and all connections airtight. The system's now ready to use. Chest cavity blood should begin collecting in the bag.

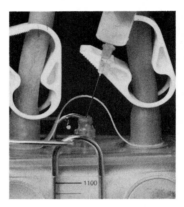

2 Add an anticoagulant, such as heparin or citrate phosphate dextrose, as ordered. Using an 18G (or smaller) needle, inject the anticoagulant through the rubber diaphragm on the collection bag's cap, as shown here.

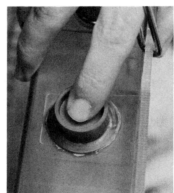

3 To collect more than one bag of blood, open a replacement bag when the first one's nearly full.
Close the clamps on top of the second bag. Before removing the first collection bag from the drainage unit, reduce excess negativity by using the high negativity relief valve. Depress the button, as shown; then release it when negativity drops to the desired level. (Watch the water seal manometer.)

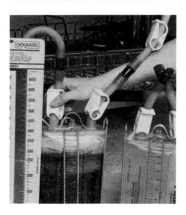

4 Close the white clamp on the patient tubing. Then, close the two white clamps on top of the collection bag, as the nurse is doing here.

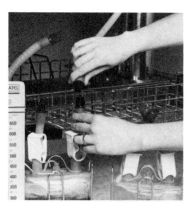

5 Disconnect all connectors on the first bag.

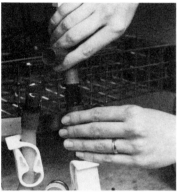

6 Remove the protective cap from the collection tubing on the replacement bag. Connect the collection tubing to the patient's chest drainage tube, using the red connectors.

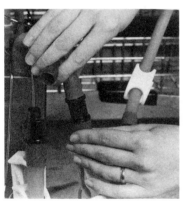

7 Now, remove the protective cap from the replacement bag's suction tube and attach the suction tube to the Pleur-evac unit, using the blue connectors. Open all clamps and inspect the system for airtight connections.

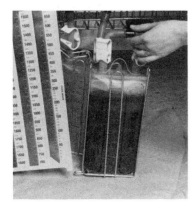

8 Attach the red (female) and blue (male) connector sections on top of the autotransfusion bag. Spread and disconnect the metal support arms, and remove the bag from the drainage unit by disconnecting the foot hook.

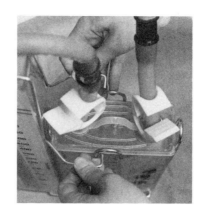

9 Then, use the foot hook and support arm to attach the replacement bag, as shown here.

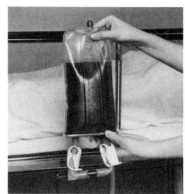

10 Now you're ready to reinfuse blood from the original collection bag. To do this, slide the bag off the support frame; then invert it so the spike port points upward.

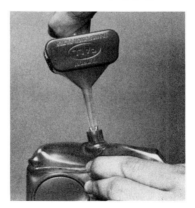

11 Remove the protective cap from the spike port and insert a microaggregate filter into the port, using a twisting motion. Prime the filter by gently squeezing the inverted bag.

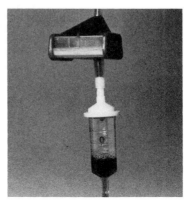

12 Continue squeezing until the filter's saturated and the drip chamber's half full, as shown here. Then, close the clamp on the reinfusion line and remove residual air from the bag. Invert the bag and suspend it from an I.V. pole; after carefully flushing the I.V. line to remove all air, infuse blood according to hospital policy.

Shock and trauma care

How to use the Receptal ATS blood collection/infusion kit

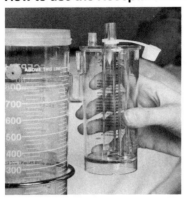

1 Your patient, who has just returned from open-heart surgery, begins bleeding uncontrollably from a mediastinal chest tube. The doctor orders autotransfusion. Here's how to connect the Receptal ATS.
   Attach the small canister (labeled Receptaseal) to the canister attachment bracket, as shown here.

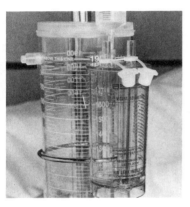

2 Inject 30 ml saline solution into the Receptaseal through the Receptaseal fill port. Fill to the minimum water level line. The water chamber now serves as both an underwater seal and an air-leak indicator. Keep the canister upright during chest drainage to eliminate leakage. (If the chamber tips over, the safety valve allows air to escape from the patient's chest while stopping air return, thus helping to prevent pneumothorax.)

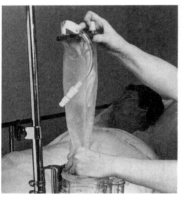

3 Using sterile technique, extend the autotransfusion liner by pulling the bottom of the liner down, as shown here. Quickly insert the liner into the large canister (labeled Receptal), keeping the thumb tab over the side port. Snap the lid on tightly so air won't leak out.

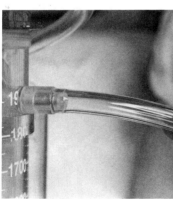

4 Now, attach the suction tubing (from a wall unit or another source) to the canister valve on the large canister's side.

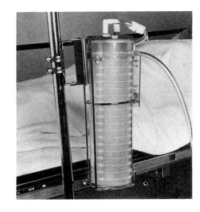

5 Turn the suction on to expand the liner in the canister. Use full suction.

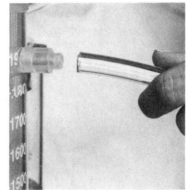

6 Disconnect the suction tubing.

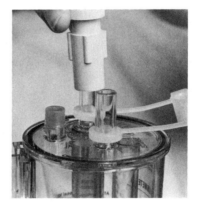

7 Then, connect the liner lid tubing to the liner lid tubing port, as the nurse is doing here.

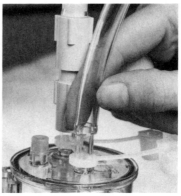

8 Connect the suction tubing to the vacuum source port on the Receptaseal, and turn on the vacuum. Because Receptaseal provides constant negative pressure of approximately 20 cm water, this system doesn't require a suction regulator or gauge. (However, if you're using either, turn it to full suction.)

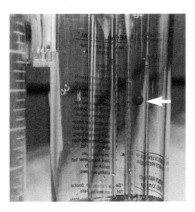

9 Check the position of the red flowmeter ball to determine if the system's receiving adequate pressure—the ball should float between the red lines, as shown here. If it doesn't rise that high, make sure the regulator or gauge is on full suction (350 mm Hg) and check for kinks or blockages in the suction tubing.

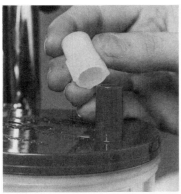

10 Next, remove the protective cap on the liner lid's patient port, using sterile technique.

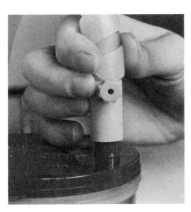

11 Connect the patient's drainage tubing to the liner lid's patient port.

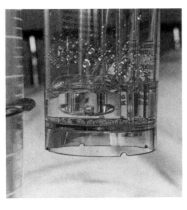

12 Make sure the patient's drainage tubing is unclamped. The system's now ready to use. Throughout the drainage procedure, check frequently for bubbling in the canister; bubbling will continue until air has emptied completely from the thoracic cavity and collection container. If bubbling doesn't stop by then, check for a leak within the entire system (including the patient).

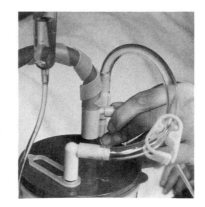

13 If the doctor has ordered an anticoagulant, such as citrate phosphate dextrose, connect the anticoagulant tubing to the anticoagulant port on the patient tubing, as shown here. If you're not using an anticoagulant, make sure the anticoagulant connector's cap remains in place.
Start the anticoagulant infusion, regulating the flow rate as ordered.

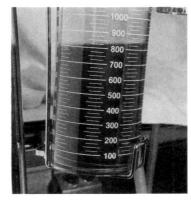

14 Monitor the patient as blood aspirated from his chest collects in the sterile liner. When about 500 to 1,000 ml of blood has collected, you're ready to begin the transfusion.

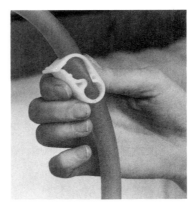

15 Prepare for the transfusion by clamping the patient tubing and the anticoagulant tubing close to the canister. *Caution:* Always clamp the patient's line before turning off the suction or disconnecting any part of the suction line. Otherwise, pneumothorax may result.

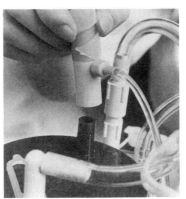

16 Then, stop the anticoagulant infusion and disconnect the patient line (which includes the anticoagulant connector) from the liner lid's patient port.

Shock and trauma care

How to use the Receptal ATS blood collection/infusion kit continued

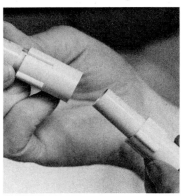

17 Clamp the liner lid tubing and disconnect the tubing from the Receptaseal. Remove the sterile spacer from the liner lid tubing, as shown here.

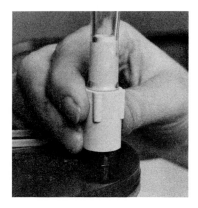

18 Immediately connect the liner lid tubing to the patient port, as shown here. Secure the connection by giving the tubing a hard push and twist.

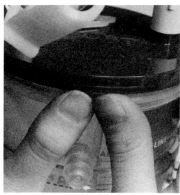

19 Remove the liner by pressing against the lid's thumb tab.

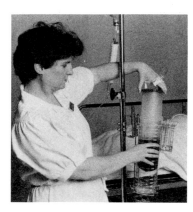

20 Remove the liner from the canister and squeeze out the air. If you plan to continue blood collection, replace the liner with a sterile one. Reconnect the patient and suction lines, as already shown.

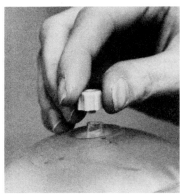

21 To prepare for the transfusion, invert the blood bag and remove the cap on the spike port.

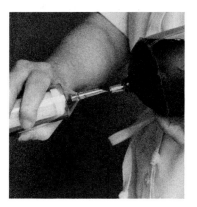

22 Pull out the spike port and close the clamp on the blood bag tubing. To insert the microaggregate filter, hold the bag in the crook of your arm, as the nurse is doing here. Placing the filter's spike into the bag's spike port, use a pushing and twisting motion to pierce the bag's diaphragm. Keep the filter level with the spike port.

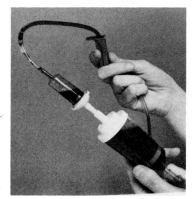

23 Next, open the clamp and keep it open. Invert the blood bag and squeeze it forcefully until the blood reaches the halfway mark on the filter's drip chamber. Then, close the clamp.

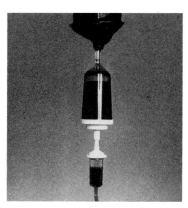

24 Hang the bag from the I.V. pole and flush the tubing to remove all air. Attach the blood bag tubing to the patient's I.V. tubing, open the clamp, and begin the transfusion.

Preventing autotransfusion complications

Despite advantages, autotransfusion can cause complications. To avoid problems, follow the guidelines below.

To prevent embolism:
• Check the entire system for air leaks before reinfusing blood.
• Use extra in-line micropore filters.
• Administer corticosteroids, as ordered, when performing massive autotransfusion.

To prevent hemolysis:
• Keep the suction device tip below the blood's surface (preferably at the bottom of the blood pool) to decrease blood-air contact.
• Limit suction pressure to 15 mm Hg.
• Try to prevent acidosis, dehydration, and shock.

To prevent sepsis:
• Don't reinfuse shed blood that's been stored for more than 4 hours.
• Never add autotransfusion blood to the donor pool (autotransfusion blood can't be stored).
• Use in-line micropore filters to trap contaminants.
• Don't perform autotransfusion if you know or suspect that your patient has a systemic or cardiopulmonary infection, a cancerous lesion in the hemorrhage area, or a thoracoabdominal injury with possible intestinal contamination; or if he has any signs or symptoms of GI tract disruption.
• If you suspect your patient may be developing an infection, give broad-spectrum systemic antibiotics, as ordered.
• Never use the same autotransfusion device for two patients. Discard the entire device when your patient no longer needs it.

To prevent coagulopathy:
• Add an anticoagulant, such as citrate phosphate dextrose, as ordered.
• Try to avoid transfusing more than 4,000 ml blood. If you must transfuse more, supplement it with fresh-frozen plasma and platelets, as ordered.

To prevent equipment malfunction:
• Don't let furniture, bed linens, or other items block the autotransfusion device's atmospheric vent.
• When using the Receptal ATS, check for drainage overflow into the Receptaseal canister. If overflow occurs, replace the Receptaseal canister to prevent valve malfunction.

Using the Morgan Therapeutic Lens

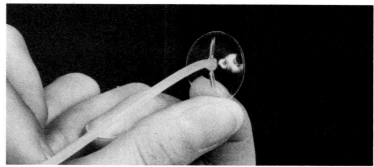

If your patient has a serious eye injury or infection, she may need immediate ocular lavage and medication to prevent permanent eye damage or complications. Inserted early, the Morgan Therapeutic Lens shown above minimizes damage and promotes healing. For many patients, it also relieves pain immediately. By providing continuous irrigation, it eliminates the need for repeated drop instillation.

The Morgan lens consists of a molded scleral lens that connects to a 6"-long silicone tube. One end of the tube attaches to a small, central hole in the lens; the other end, to a molded Luer-Lok adapter that you'll connect to a syringe or an I.V. line. Fluid and medication, which flow through the tube at a controlled rate, can be stopped or changed without lens removal. The lens stays securely in place and flow remains constant even if the patient's moved.

Before ocular surgery, the doctor may use the Morgan lens to flush the patient's conjunctiva. During eyelid surgery, he may use it to protect and irrigate the eye.

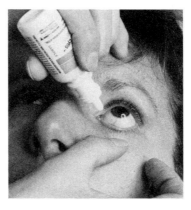

1 First, instill a topical anesthetic, as the nurse is doing here.

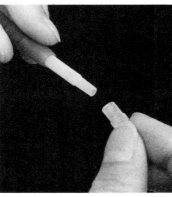

2 To provide continuous lavage, attach the lens tube's adapter to an I.V. set containing the ordered solution. Then, begin the flow at the ordered rate. *Note:* You can also use a syringe to irrigate the eye.

Shock and trauma care

Using the Morgan Therapeutic Lens continued

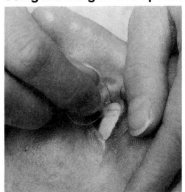

3 Next, ask the patient to look down, as shown here. Insert the edge of the lens under her upper lid. Then tell her to look up as you retract her lower lid.

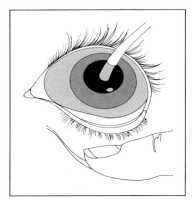

4 Release the lower lid over the lens. Securely in place, the lens now irrigates the eye continuously.

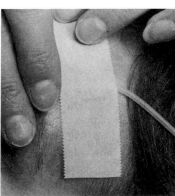

5 To prevent accidental lens displacement, tape the tube to the patient's forehead. Wipe off any excess solution with a towel.

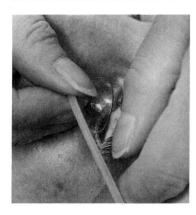

6 To remove the lens, ask the patient to look up as you retract the lower lid from the lens' lower border. Then, while holding this position, have the patient look down. Retract her upper lid and slide the lens out, as shown here.

Morgan Therapeutic Lens: Treatment guidelines

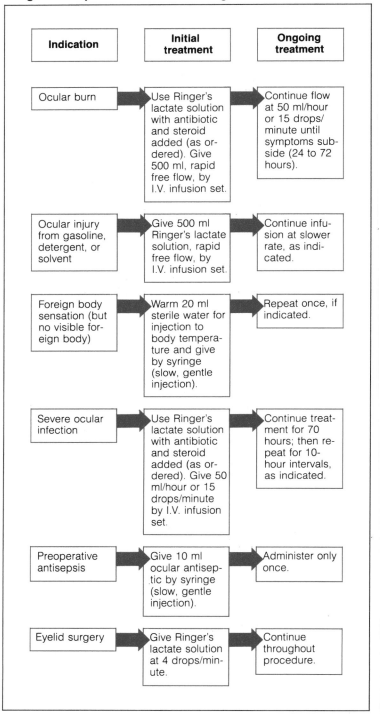

Indication	Initial treatment	Ongoing treatment
Ocular burn	Use Ringer's lactate solution with antibiotic and steroid added (as ordered). Give 500 ml, rapid free flow, by I.V. infusion set.	Continue flow at 50 ml/hour or 15 drops/minute until symptoms subside (24 to 72 hours).
Ocular injury from gasoline, detergent, or solvent	Give 500 ml Ringer's lactate solution, rapid free flow, by I.V. infusion set.	Continue infusion at slower rate, as indicated.
Foreign body sensation (but no visible foreign body)	Warm 20 ml sterile water for injection to body temperature and give by syringe (slow, gentle injection).	Repeat once, if indicated.
Severe ocular infection	Use Ringer's lactate solution with antibiotic and steroid added (as ordered). Give 50 ml/hour or 15 drops/minute by I.V. infusion set.	Continue treatment for 70 hours; then repeat for 10-hour intervals, as indicated.
Preoperative antisepsis	Give 10 ml ocular antiseptic by syringe (slow, gentle injection).	Administer only once.
Eyelid surgery	Give Ringer's lactate solution at 4 drops/minute.	Continue throughout procedure.

Burn care

Skillful application of new therapies and products improves the prognosis for many burn victims. In the next few pages, you'll learn about experimental skin coverings under development and about new dressing techniques that limit the progress of burn injuries and promote healing. For example, you'll learn how to:
• apply a Sulfamylon sandwich, a layered dressing that protects a burn with lower (and less irritating) Sulfamylon concentrations than you applied in the past.
• use E-Z Derm Temporary Skin Substitute, a unique xenograft that acts as a temporary second skin during the healing process.
• apply Water-Jel, a one-step emergency burn dressing that immediately eases pain and limits burn damage.

UPDATE

Burn care: New skin coverings

Two experimental techniques may soon provide coverings for burned tissue without depleting a burn victim's scarce supply of undamaged skin.
• *Cultured epithelium.* From seed cells originating with a stamp-sized specimen of the patient's own tissue, researchers have cultured sheets of epidermal cells capable of covering an area 10,000 times greater than the original tissue specimen. After placement over the wound, these cells continue to replicate, covering the wound in about 3 months. Reasonably durable, the graft may remain supple for up to 2 years; however, some patients experience wound contraction or blistering.

• *Artificial skin.* A composite skin graft incorporating an artificial dermal layer and an epidermal autograft can cover large burn areas; however, this technique still requires harvesting from the patient's limited tissue supply. A collagen matrix created from animal tissue serves as a dermal layer over the wound; a thin Silastic sheet serves as the epidermis. After the matrix vascularizes, the doctor peels away the Silastic sheet and replaces it with an epidermal autograft. By refining techniques for impregnating the artificial matrix with cultured epidermal cells from the patient's own tissue, researchers may eventually eliminate the need to harvest large amounts of donor tissue.

Using a Sulfamylon sandwich for better burn care

An antimicrobial, 11.2% mafenide acetate cream (Sulfamylon) prevents burn wound infection. But it has several drawbacks: it's severely painful to apply and remove, and it inhibits graft tissue healing.

To solve these problems, burn specialists have developed a layered dressing that eliminates most adverse effects while still guarding against infection. Called a Sulfamylon sandwich, this dressing bathes the wound in an aqueous solution containing lower Sulfamylon concentrations (0.6% to 1.2%). Virtually painless to apply, the dressing can be changed at bedside without painful hydrotherapy—and without disturbing underlying skin grafts. The photostory on the following page shows how to apply it.

As ordered, change the dressing's outer two layers after 12 hours. Change the entire dressing after 72 hours.

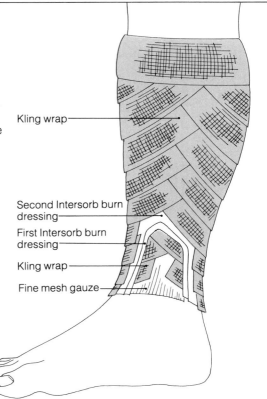

Kling wrap

Second Intersorb burn dressing

First Intersorb burn dressing

Kling wrap

Fine mesh gauze

Burn care

How to apply a Sulfamylon sandwich

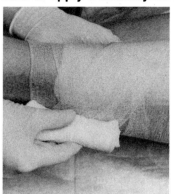

1 Soak fine-mesh gauze in warm normal saline solution. Apply one layer over the burn. Then apply a single layer of Kling wrap soaked in normal saline solution over the first layer, wrapping in a figure-eight pattern, as shown. *Caution:* Don't wrap too tightly; if the dressing dries out, the Kling wrap could shrink and cut off circulation.

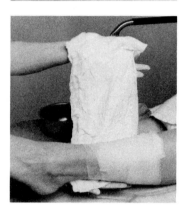

2 Soak an Intersorb burn dressing (a multilayered coarse-mesh gauze pad) with normal saline solution, and coat it with Sulfamylon. Then place the dressing over the Kling wrap. Center it over the wound, not over healed skin.

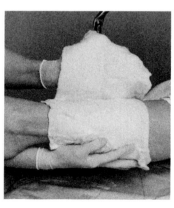

3 Soak another Intersorb dressing in normal saline solution, and put it over the Sulfamylon-coated dressing.

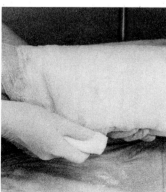

4 Secure the Sulfamylon sandwich with Kling wrap; then soak the entire dressing with sterile normal saline solution.

To prevent drying, soak the entire dressing in normal saline solution every 6 hours.

E-Z Derm Temporary Skin Substitute: An advance in burn care

You're on duty in the emergency department when Joan Norris, age 29, seeks treatment for a scald on her forearm, which she injured while cooking. The doctor administers a local anesthetic and debrides blisters, revealing a partial-thickness wound. As ordered, you dress the wound with E-Z Derm Temporary Skin Substitute (see following photostory).

A porcine xenograft, Genetic Laboratories' E-Z Derm is a biosynthetic dressing that acts as a temporary second skin until the patient's own skin regenerates. Antigenically inert, it remains in place over an uncomplicated burn until healing's complete. (Contaminated or chronic wounds may require frequent E-Z Derm changes.) E-Z Derm with Silver provides antimicrobial protection without the painful dressing changes required to apply silver sulfadiazine cream.

To maximize E-Z Derm adherence, the wound must be thoroughly debrided beforehand. As the wound heals, the dressing separates from it. *Note:* If the wound involves several tissue depths, the E-Z Derm may separate from some areas sooner than others. Simply trim off the separated portions to prevent snagging.

The doctor may order E-Z Derm for partial- or full-thickness burns, skin graft sites, and ulcers (Stages II through IV). E-Z Derm can also help him determine whether a full-thickness burn is ready to receive an autograft.

Because most patients don't need frequent dressing changes, E-Z Derm saves you time and helps reduce hospital stays. In addition, it:
• reduces pain and the risk of bacterial contamination
• controls fluid and heat loss
• promotes early tissue granulation
• promotes homeostasis.

You can store E-Z Derm for 1 year at room temperature. For convenience, it's available in perforated and unperforated patches and in sheets and rolls. (Perforated E-Z Derm permits exudate transudation.)

Caution: Patients sensitive to porcine products, silver, or sulfa drugs, and those with serum allergies, shouldn't use E-Z Derm.

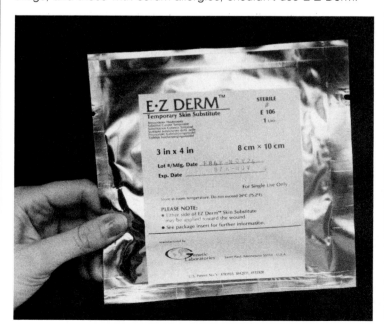

Applying E-Z Derm Temporary Skin Substitute

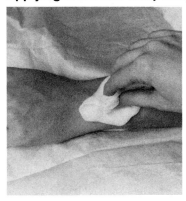

1 Obtain the ordered E-Z Derm (with or without silver; perforated or unperforated), sterile gloves, and sterile gauze wrap or flexible net dressing.

Explain the procedure to the patient. Then cleanse the wound thoroughly, removing all traces of drainage and topical medication, if present. *Important:* The wound must be completely debrided and cleansed to maximize E-Z Derm adherence.

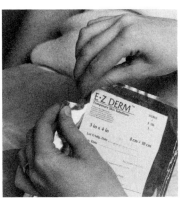

2 Open the E-Z Derm package, using aseptic technique.

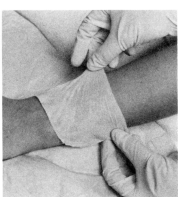

3 Don gloves and remove the E-Z Derm patch from its gauze liner (discard the liner). Place it directly on the wound (either side will adhere), as shown here. Cover the wound completely and make sure the dressing lies smoothly over the wound. (If you need more than one dressing to cover the wound, overlap them slightly.)

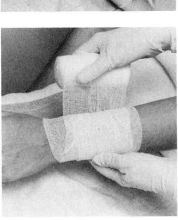

4 Secure the E-Z Derm patch with gauze wrap. (If you applied a perforated E-Z Derm patch, moisten the gauze.)

While the wound heals, monitor the patient for signs of infection: fever, drainage, and E-Z Derm nonadherence. Also assess for an allergic reaction. If your patient's going home with E-Z Derm, teach him to care for it (see the box at right).

PATIENT TEACHING

Teaching your patient to care for E-Z Derm

If your patient goes home with E-Z Derm Temporary Skin Substitute, you'll want to teach him how to care for the wound and dressing. Cover the following points.

What to expect:
• After 3 to 4 hours, the wound may feel tight, but it shouldn't hurt, burn, or itch.
• Within 24 hours, E-Z Derm adheres (clings) to the wound.
• While the wound heals, E-Z Derm may change color.
• At 5 to 7 days, E-Z Derm may become dry and look like a scab.
• At 8 to 11 days, E-Z Derm separates from the wound. The healed skin looks pink.

How to care for your wound:
• Keep the wound area still for 5 hours after E-Z Derm's application; then limit movement the first 24 hours. After 24 hours, continue normal activity and exercise, as prescribed by your doctor.
• Don't remove E-Z Derm unless your doctor tells you to do so.
• Keep it dry for 24 hours. After that, you may bathe normally if you don't immerse it for more than 5 minutes.
• Reapply gauze, as instructed by your doctor.
• When E-Z Derm begins to separate from the wound, trim its stiff edges with clean scissors.

Call your doctor if:
• you have a fever.
• you have pain.
• your E-Z Derm patch doesn't cling to the wound after 24 hours.
• pus forms under it or the wound seems weepy.
• you notice redness around the wound that wasn't there before.

Burn care

Water-Jel: Emergency therapy at the scene

A one-step emergency dressing, Water-Jel combines 100% new wool dressing material with a bacteriostatic, biodegradable, water-soluble gel containing natural oils. Available in a variety of sizes (from a 2" × 2" pad to an 8' × 6' heat shield), Water-Jel products can simultaneously extinguish flames and begin primary burn treatment. They're not toxic or irritating to the eyes.

When applied to a burn, Water-Jel:
- *reduces or eliminates pain by coating exposed nerve endings and protecting them from irritating air currents.*
- *lowers skin temperature and absorbs heat. Because it lowers skin temperature by heat transference, not evaporation, it won't induce hypothermia.*
- *reduces infection risk. The bacteriostatic gel protects injured tissue from airborne microbes.*
- *facilitates medical care by softening burned clothes and preventing them from adhering to wounds. Because it's water-soluble, Water-Jel washes off with sterile water or saline solution.*

After applying Water-Jel (see following photostory), leave it in place for at least 20 minutes. If necessary, you can leave it in place for 8 hours, until secondary medical care becomes available.

Special considerations
You can use Water-Jel for any burn type, with these precautions:
- *Before treating an electrical burn victim, eliminate the power source to protect victim and rescuer from shocks.*
- *To treat chemical burns, follow the chemical manufacturer's instructions; for example, wipe off the chemical and flood the burn with water. Then apply Water-Jel. Caution: Don't use Water-Jel to treat burns caused by water-reactive chemicals, or it may extend the burn area.*

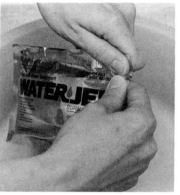

1 Tear open the foil packet at the precut notches. (Don't apply any Water-Jel product to a burn if the packet has previously been opened. You can still use the product to extinguish flames, however.)

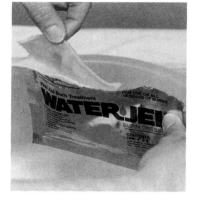

2 Remove the dressing from the packet, avoiding unnecessary handling.

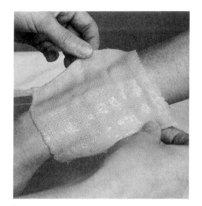

3 If clothing has melted over the wound, apply Water-Jel over the clothing—the solution will soak through clothing to treat the burn. However, if you can quickly and easily remove the clothing, do so. Apply the dressing loosely, without pressure. *Note:* For extensive burns, use a Water-Jel blanket or heat shield (see following photostory).

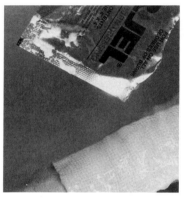

4 If solution remains in the packet, pour it onto the dressing.

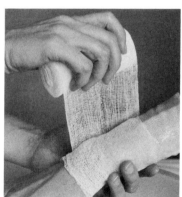

5 Secure the dressing with gauze or any other available bandaging material to keep it in place during transport.

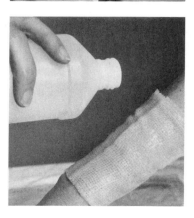

6 To remove Water-Jel for secondary burn treatment, wash it off with sterile water or normal saline solution.

Using a Water-Jel blanket or heat shield

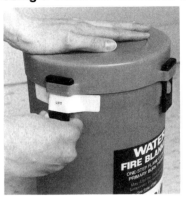

1 To remove a large Water-Jel product (a blanket or heat shield) from its canister, hold the canister upright. With a quick snapping motion, break the paper seals on one of the plastic clips. Pull the clip out and away from its catch.

Repeat the action to remove all four clips.

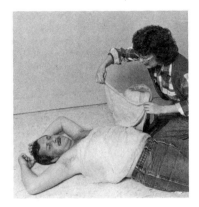

4 If melted clothes cover the victim's burned skin, simply apply the blanket over the clothing. The Water-Jel solution will soak through to the skin. However, if you can quickly and easily remove clothing, do so.

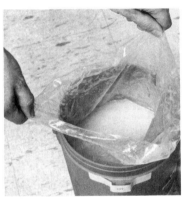

2 Pull up on the sealed plastic bag. (You can't remove it because it's attached to the canister's inside.) Then grasp the bag on each side and tear it open along its sealed top, as shown. Or cut the bag open with scissors, if available.

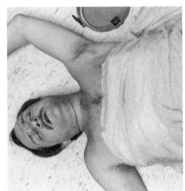

5 Depending on the burn's location and size, loosely wrap the blanket around the victim or lay it on top of the burn. (If the victim's clothes are burning, the blanket will extinguish the fire and begin first aid in one step.)

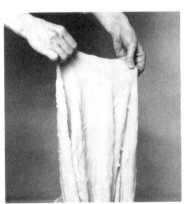

3 Remove the blanket from the bag. To minimize contamination, handle it as little as possible and don't let it touch the ground.

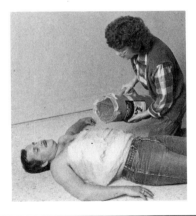

6 Pour any Water-Jel solution remaining in the plastic bag onto the blanket. To keep the blanket in place during transport, loosely secure it with any available bandaging material.

QUESTIONS & ANSWERS

Questions about Water-Jel

If you've never used Water-Jel products before, you may have the following questions. The manufacturer, Trilling Resources, Ltd., supplies the answers.

Q. *How long can Water-Jel be stored?*
A. Water-Jel burn dressings have a 3-year shelf life, as do nylon-packaged products. The Water-Jel blanket and other products packaged in canisters have a 3-year medical shelf life, with an additional 2 years as firefighting equipment. A canister product's life as firefighting equipment can last 2 more years if it's refurbished with Water-Jel refurbishing jel.

Q. *Do temperature extremes affect the product's effectiveness?*
A. No. The product remains effective after freezing and thawing and after exposure to extreme heat and humidity.

Q. *Can I use a product more than once?*
A. You can use each product only once as a medical device, but larger products can be refurbished and reused repeatedly as firefighting devices.

Q. *How do I dispose of a product after use?*
A. You can dispose of it in any convenient way—it's biodegradable and nontoxic.

Digoxin overdose

Potentially fatal, severe digoxin intoxication requires immediate treatment. Digibind (digoxin immune Fab [Ovine]) can quickly reverse the condition. You may also give it to treat life-threatening digitoxin intoxication.

Read these three pages to learn more about this important new drug. You'll learn:
• how to recognize digoxin toxicity
• how Digibind fits into the treatment protocol for digoxin toxicity
• how to estimate dosage, based on the degree of digoxin toxicity and the patient's weight
• what precautions to take before and during Digibind administration.

Digibind: New treatment for digoxin toxicity

A powder of antigen-binding agents derived from sheep antibodies, Digibind binds with digoxin molecules and prevents them from binding at receptor sites in the body—thus reversing digoxin's toxic effects. Digibind/digoxin complexes accumulate in the blood for excretion by the kidneys.

Indications and precautions

As ordered, give Digibind to treat severe digoxin intoxication (see the treatment protocol on the opposite page). In cases of overdose by ingestion, these amounts cause severe intoxication and may trigger cardiac arrest: more than 10 mg in previously healthy adults; more than 4 mg in previously healthy children. A steady-state serum concentration greater than 2.5 ng/ml indicates toxicity; a concentration greater than 10 ng/ml may cause cardiac arrest. *Important:* Rising serum potassium concentrations induced by digoxin overdose may indicate impending cardiac arrest. Give Digibind if the patient's potassium concentration exceeds 5 mEq/liter.

No known contraindications to Digibind exist, and you can give it to children and infants if indicated.

No allergic or febrile reactions to Digibind have been reported. As a precaution, however, keep emergency drugs and equipment at hand in case anaphylaxis develops.

Note: Digibind has also successfully treated digitoxin overdose.

Dosage and administration

Dosage (measured in 40-mg vials) depends on the amount of digoxin to be neutralized. The average patient needs about 10 vials (400 mg). See the charts on page 46 for dosage guidelines.

If the doctor can't estimate the amount of digoxin ingested, he may order up to 20 vials, which can safely reverse toxic effects in both adults and children. (Closely monitor a child for fluid overload.) If necessary, the doctor may order another dose (based on the patient's condition) after several hours. *Important:* If the patient fails to respond to Digibind, reassess for other possible causes of his symptoms.

In most circumstances, give Digibind I.V. over 30 minutes, preferably through a 0.22-micron membrane filter. If cardiac arrest seems imminent, however, give a bolus injection.

Nursing considerations

• If possible, obtain serum digoxin levels before beginning Digibind therapy. Remember, however, that interpreting lab results may be difficult, especially if the patient took his last digoxin dose a short time earlier: serum and tissue concentrations don't reach equilibrium for 6 to 8 hours. After Digibind administration, serum digoxin levels rise precipitously, but most serum digoxin is bound with Digibind and therefore can't bind with receptor sites. Consequently, serum digoxin levels won't accurately reflect response to therapy. Let the patient's clinical condition guide treatment. *Note:* In acute ingestion overdose, try to ascertain (from the patient, a relative, or a friend) how much he swallowed.
• To reconstitute the drug, gently mix each vial's contents with 4 ml sterile water for injection. (If ordered, dilute the reconstituted drug to a convenient volume with sterile isotonic saline solution.) Use the reconstituted drug immediately, or refrigerate it for up to 4 hours.
• Monitor the patient for hyperkalemia and hypokalemia. Digoxin intoxication causes potassium to shift from cells to the blood, causing high serum potassium levels with a total body potassium deficit. After treatment with Digibind, potassium shifts back into cells and hypokalemia may develop rapidly.
• Closely monitor patients with intrinsically poor cardiac function for problems related to withdrawal of digoxin's inotropic effects. If necessary, the doctor may order dopamine, dobutamine, or a vasodilator.
• Don't resume digoxin therapy until Digibind has been eliminated from the body—several days for most patients. Patients with impaired renal function may need a week or more.

Digoxin intoxication: Danger signs

Digoxin has a narrow therapeutic range. For some patients, even a conservative therapeutic dose can be toxic. Of course, this explains why toxicity from digoxin and other cardiac glycosides (digitoxin, deslanoside, digitalis leaf) is relatively common.

A patient who's also taking certain other drugs, or who has certain disorders, faces a particularly high risk of toxicity. Risk factors include reduced renal or hepatic function, electrolyte imbalance, myocardial infarction, pulmonary disease, hypothyroidism, and concurrent quinidine or verapamil therapy.

Closely monitor patients taking digoxin for these signs and symptoms of toxicity.

Cardiac dysrhythmias:
● Premature ventricular contractions (unifocal and multifocal)
● Ventricular bigeminy or trigeminy
● Ventricular tachycardia
● Sinoatrial exit block or arrest
● Second-degree atrioventricular (AV) block (Type I)
● Third-degree AV block
● Atrial fibrillation with slow ventricular rate
● Accelerated nonparoxysmal AV junctional rhythms
● Atrial tachycardia with AV block

Other:
● Worsening congestive heart failure
● Hypotension
● Fatigue, weakness
● Vision disturbances (halos, blurred vision, light flashes, photophobia, diplopia)
● Nausea, vomiting
● Anorexia
● Abdominal pain
● Hallucinations, abnormal dreams
● Dizziness
● Headache
● Diarrhea

Digoxin intoxication: Treatment protocol

Give Digibind to treat *severe* digoxin overdose only. The following protocol, based on four levels of intoxication (ranging from least to most severe), provides a standard for assessment and treatment.

LEVEL 1

● Reduce or withhold digoxin (treat on outpatient basis).

LEVEL 2

● Hospitalize patient.
● Withdraw patient from digoxin therapy.
● Treat electrolyte imbalances, acid-base disturbances, and low PO_2 levels.
● Assess for other drugs that may aggravate patient's condition: catecholamines and calcium salts; beta blockers and calcium channel blockers (in patients with AV block); and drugs that raise serum digoxin levels, such as quinidine.

LEVEL 3

● Provide drug and pacemaker therapy to correct dysrhythmias.
● Administer Digibind if necessary.

LEVEL 4

● Administer Digibind immediately to treat massive digoxin overdose.

Digoxin overdose

Single-ingestion overdose: Dosage guidelines

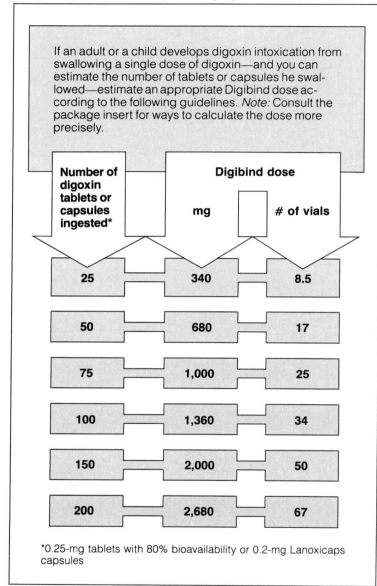

If an adult or a child develops digoxin intoxication from swallowing a single dose of digoxin—and you can estimate the number of tablets or capsules he swallowed—estimate an appropriate Digibind dose according to the following guidelines. *Note:* Consult the package insert for ways to calculate the dose more precisely.

Number of digoxin tablets or capsules ingested*	Digibind dose	
	mg	# of vials
25	340	8.5
50	680	17
75	1,000	25
100	1,360	34
150	2,000	50
200	2,680	67

*0.25-mg tablets with 80% bioavailability or 0.2-mg Lanoxicaps capsules

Estimating dosage based on serum digoxin levels

Guidelines for adults

If you know an adult patient's *steady-state* serum digoxin concentration, estimate the Digibind dose based on the patient's weight. Use this color-coded chart as a guide. (The dose is expressed in number of vials.)

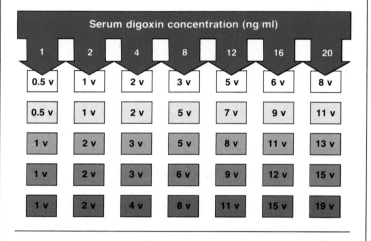

| Patient weight (kg) | 40 | 60 | 70 | 80 | 100 |

Serum digoxin concentration (ng/ml)						
1	2	4	8	12	16	20
0.5 v	1 v	2 v	3 v	5 v	6 v	8 v
0.5 v	1 v	2 v	5 v	7 v	9 v	11 v
1 v	2 v	3 v	5 v	8 v	11 v	13 v
1 v	2 v	3 v	6 v	9 v	12 v	15 v
1 v	2 v	4 v	8 v	11 v	15 v	19 v

Guidelines for infants and children

For an infant, reconstitute a 40-mg vial, as directed, and deliver the dose with a tuberculin syringe. To give a very small dose (2 mg or less), dilute a reconstituted vial with 36 ml sterile isotonic saline solution to create a 1-mg/ml concentration.

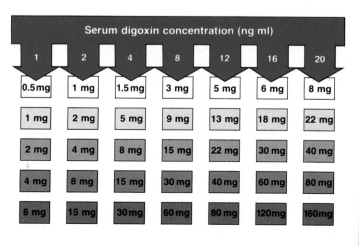

| Patient weight (kg) | 1 | 3 | 5 | 10 | 20 |

Serum digoxin concentration (ng/ml)						
1	2	4	8	12	16	20
0.5 mg	1 mg	1.5 mg	3 mg	5 mg	6 mg	8 mg
1 mg	2 mg	5 mg	9 mg	13 mg	18 mg	22 mg
2 mg	4 mg	8 mg	15 mg	22 mg	30 mg	40 mg
4 mg	8 mg	15 mg	30 mg	40 mg	60 mg	80 mg
8 mg	15 mg	30 mg	60 mg	80 mg	120 mg	160 mg

Caring for the
Medical/Surgical
Patient

| A.I.D.S. | Diabetes | Drug therapy | I.V. therapy |
| Cancer | Diagnostic tests | Medication administration | Postoperative care |

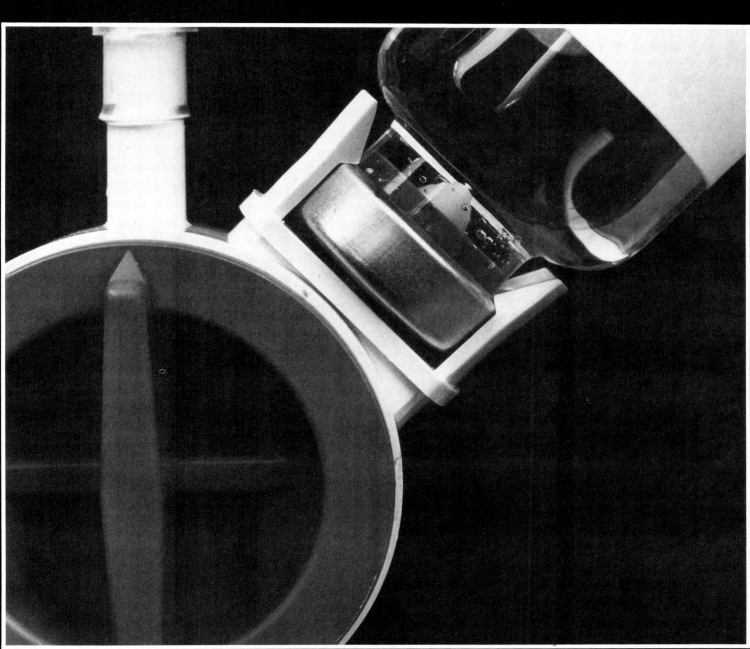

A.I.D.S.

Few diseases inspire quite the same emotions as acquired immune deficiency syndrome (AIDS). Besides coping with a terminal illness, its victims may have to deal with rejection by friends and family members who fear the disease. As a nurse, you know that AIDS doesn't spread by casual contact—yet you may unwittingly contribute to a patient's emotional isolation with fears of your own.

To date, no health care worker has contracted AIDS from patient contact. You can protect yourself from unnecessary risk—and eliminate unreasonable fears—by following the recommended infection control precautions detailed in this section. Also use this information to teach your patients about AIDS—how it spreads, who's at risk, and how it's treated.

UPDATE

AIDS update

Characterized by a deficiency in cell-mediated immunity (T cell immunity), AIDS leaves its victims susceptible to infections and cancers that healthy people normally resist. The responsible organism: retrovirus HIV (human immunodeficiency virus). *Note:* Other names for this virus include human T-cell lymphotropic virus, type III (HTLV-III) and lymphadenopathy-associated virus (LAV).

Present in an infected person's blood, semen, and other body fluids, the virus may spread during sexual intercourse or during transfusion of contaminated blood or blood products. It can also spread transplacentally, from an infected woman to her unborn child.

In the United States, most AIDS victims fall into one or more of these groups:
- homosexual or bisexual men
- intravenous drug users
- hemophiliacs (and others who've received blood transfusions)
- heterosexual partners of infected people
- children born to infected women.

The Centers for Disease Control (CDC) recognizes a similar disorder called AIDS-related complex (ARC). Patients with ARC test positive for HIV without having developed the opportunistic infections or cancers characteristic of AIDS. However, many of these patients eventually develop AIDS.

Signs and symptoms

Patients with AIDS typically report these symptoms: fever, weight loss, diarrhea, night sweats, fatigue, and/or lymphadenopathy. (Many ARC patients also experience these symptoms.) However, some AIDS patients remain asymptomatic until they develop an opportunistic infection or Kaposi's sarcoma (KS), a purplish, palpable, usually painless skin cancer that develops almost exclusively in patients with cell-

mediated immune deficiencies. AIDS-related opportunistic infections include *Pneumocystis carinii* pneumonia (the most common), *Candida albicans* stomatitis, *Toxoplasma gondii* encephalitis, cytomegalovirus, and parasitic infections.

An AIDS patients under medical care may experience a pattern of illness and remission lasting 8 months to 2 years. Between illnesses, he may feel healthy. Eventually, however, an infection or malignancy will kill him.

An infected child may develop AIDS after an incubation period of 5 to 11 months. Besides KS and the opportunistic infections already mentioned, he may develop chronic diffuse interstitial pneumonitis and enlarged parotid glands.

Diagnosis

Diagnosis rests on the patient's symptoms and a positive test for HIV antibody. The test, enzyme-linked immunosorbent assay (ELISA), is always repeated when it's positive; results are confirmed by the western blot analysis, a more specific antibody test. (Blood banks now use the ELISA test to screen blood and blood products for AIDS contamination.)

A person who tests positive for HIV antibody has been infected with the AIDS virus. Although he may not have AIDS, he's considered capable of transmitting the disease through blood and sexual contact.

HIV can also be cultured from an infected person's cells. While this slow and difficult test isn't used for routine diagnoses, it's useful for evaluating the effectiveness of experimental drugs.

Other diagnostic tests for AIDS include:
- a complete blood count with differential to check for lymphocytopenia
- an immune profile

- skin testing with common antigens to evaluate cell-mediated immunity.

Treatment

No cure for AIDS exists yet, but several drugs look promising. Azidothymidine (AZT) appears to arrest HIV's ability to reproduce. Available in oral form, it causes fewer adverse effects than many other drugs under study.

Adverse effects linked to AZT include headache, rash, anemia, leukopenia, and granulocytopenia. About 25% of patients receiving AZT during one study required blood transfusions after 4 to 8 weeks of therapy. Other drugs undergoing clinical trials include suramin, ribavirin, interferon A, and HPA-23.

Aside from such drugs, AIDS treatment is primarily supportive, aimed at curing or controlling complications as they develop.

Your role

Closely monitor the patient for early signs of complications. Frequently assess his respiratory, neurologic, nutritional, and skin status, as well as bowel and urinary function. Also teach him how to care for himself and how to avoid transmitting the virus to others (see the information on the following page).

When caring for an AIDS patient:
- provide emotional support. Besides facing death, he must deal with social disapproval, a changed body image, and possibly a loss of support by family and friends. He may also lose his job and health insurance.
- encourage him to eat well, exercise as his condition permits, and maintain good hygiene.
- teach him how to minimize infection risk, how to recognize infections and cancers, and what to do when they develop.
- refer him and those close to him to a support group or counselor.

What to tell your patients about AIDS

Today, just about anyone who's sexually active and who has more than one sex partner could be considered at risk for AIDS. The same goes for drug users who share drug paraphernalia. To slow the disease's spread, educate the public about the disease and how to avoid it. Follow these guidelines, based on U.S. Public Health Service recommendations.

For all sexually active people:	• During sexual activity, use a condom to protect both partners from contact with body fluids (semen, blood, vaginal fluids, and urine) and feces. • Avoid sex with multiple partners. Also avoid sex with those who have multiple partners, such as prostitutes. • Practice conservative sex. Avoid oral-genital contact, anal intercourse, and any practice that may injure tissue.
For injectable drug users:	• Never share needles or syringes. • Don't donate blood, plasma, sperm, or any body tissue.
For people in other high-risk groups, including male homosexuals:	• Seek regular medical evaluation. • Don't donate blood, plasma, sperm, or any body tissue. • (For women) Take the HIV antibody test before becoming pregnant. Avoid pregnancy if you test positive or if you're at risk of contracting AIDS during pregnancy—you could transmit the disease to the infant.
For those who test positive for HIV:	Take the precautions recommended for members of high-risk groups. In addition: • Inform past, present, or prospective sex partners, and anyone you may have shared a needle with, that you tested positive. Encourage them to seek counseling and testing. • Inform your doctor, dentist, and eye doctor of your positive HIV status so they can take precautions. • Don't share toothbrushes, razors, or other items that might be contaminated with blood. • Use bleach to clean blood or other body fluids spilled on household surfaces, using 1 part bleach to 10 parts water. (Avoid skin contact with the bleach.)

Children with AIDS: Dealing with chronic problems

As AIDS spreads in the general population, it claims more and more children among its victims. Most of these children contracted the disease prenatally from women who have AIDS or who test positive for HIV antibodies.

Women who may have AIDS or who may have been exposed to the HIV virus should undergo testing before becoming pregnant and should postpone pregnancy if they test positive. Those at risk include prostitutes and women who use illicit I.V. drugs, live in a country where heterosexual transmission is common, or have had sex with a man at high risk.

An infant who may have been infected prenatally should be tested after age 4 months. (Before that age, his B cells may be too immature for an immune response.) Because maternal antibodies may cause a false-positive result, he should be tested again at age 6 months.

If the child develops AIDS, teach the family the importance of hand washing and other infection-control techniques. Encourage them to wear gloves during diaper changes. Tell them to talk to the doctor about a suitable immunization program—live-virus vaccines can kill an immunodeficient child, but killed-virus vaccines provide much-needed protection. *Note:* Some doctors recommend live-virus vaccines in lower doses for AIDS victims; however, this is controversial.

A child with AIDS faces a host of debilitating and potentially fatal complications. Use the following information to provide the best possible nursing care.

Respiratory infection
• Assess the child's respiratory status and his need for supplementary oxygen (based on blood gas values).
• Give antibiotics, as ordered.
• Teach parents to recognize signs of respiratory infection and to call the doctor immediately if they occur.

Lactose intolerance
• Provide a lactose-free diet, using soy formulas instead of milk.

Malnutrition
• Give the family a detailed nutrition plan to help the child grow and gain weight normally. (He may need twice the standard Recommended Daily Allowance.)
• If lesions interfere with eating, recommend bland or soft foods served cold or at room temperature.

Diarrhea
• Instruct the family to monitor stools and to encourage the child to replace lost fluid by drinking plenty of liquids.

Protecting yourself: CDC guidelines

So far, no one has reported AIDS transmission to a health care worker during patient care, and the CDC doesn't recommend routine HIV antibody testing for health care workers who care for AIDS patients. Nevertheless, to minimize risks, you should take some precautions during any procedure that might bring you in contact with the patient's body fluids. Follow these guidelines, based on CDC recommendations.
• Initiate blood and body fluid precautions, according to hospital policy.
• Wash your hands before and after contact with the patient or any soiled items.
• Don't handle patient care equipment or assist with invasive procedures if you have any open sores or irritated skin on your hands.
• Wear gloves when touching the patient's mucous membranes or broken skin. Remove the gloves and dispose of them before touching any other patient or equipment. If you tear a glove (for example, if a needle punctures it), change the glove and remove the offending instrument from the sterile field.
• Wear a mask and gown for any procedure that might involve splashing blood or secretions—for example, suctioning.
• Dispose of needles in a punctureproof container immediately after use. *Don't* bend, cut, recap, or break needles before disposal.
• Label laboratory specimens *Blood and body fluid precautions*. Place them in plastic bags for transport (according to hospital policy).
• Clean blood and other body fluid spills with a 1:10 solution of sodium hypochlorite 5.25% (household bleach).
• If you assist an AIDS patient during childbirth, handle the infant with gloves until amniotic fluid has been removed from his skin.

Cancer

Recent advances in research hold promise for millions of cancer patients. A combination of surgery and radiation can now shrink some deep-seated tumors that resist conventional therapy. Two interferon drugs, recently approved to combat a rare cancer, may soon be used to treat more common cancers, too.

Although not new, the Ommaya reservoir is now so well accepted that you're increasingly likely to have a patient with one on your unit. Besides delivering antineoplastic drugs intraventricularly, it can also deliver antibiotics for central nervous system infections (a benefit for AIDS patients who develop this complication). It can also be used to deliver analgesics, measure cerebrospinal fluid (CSF) pressure, and obtain CSF specimens. Learn more about this valuable tool on the next page.

UPDATE

 Cancer update

New antineoplastic weapons continue to improve the survival odds for many cancer patients. Promising therapies now under investigation include:

Intraoperative radiation therapy (IORT). During surgery, the doctor removes as much of the tumor as possible. Then, while shielding healthy tissue, he bombards remaining tumor tissue with a specific radiation dose—usually 6 to 10 times that delivered during standard external beam radiation therapy.

IORT has the advantage of delivering large radiation doses directly to the tumor while sparing surrounding healthy tissue. Its disadvantages:
- In many hospitals, the patient must be moved from the operating room to the radiation therapy department in the middle of surgery, thus increasing his risk of infection and other complications.
- A one-shot treatment, IORT can't be spread out over several weeks, as in conventional therapy.

Consequently, IORT use remains limited to deep-seated or previously inoperable tumors, including some tumors of the pancreas, colon, rectum, cervix, or brain.

Biological response modifiers (BRMs). A broad group of antineoplastic agents or therapies, BRMs combat cancer by altering the host's biological response to cancer cells. BRM agents include interferon, thymic factors, monoclonal antibodies (see page 60), and interleukin-2—a substance that alters the host's immune system response.

Two interferons have been approved for use against a rare cancer, hairy-cell leukemia. They may soon be approved for more common cancers, including Kaposi's sarcoma and multiple myeloma.

Interferon alfa
Available as interferon alfa-2a, recombinant (Roferon-A) and interferon alfa-2b, recombinant (Intron A)
Indication
- Hairy-cell leukemia in patients age 18 and older
Dosage
For interferon alfa-2a
Induction dosage: 3 million IU daily for 16 to 24 weeks, subcutaneously or I.M.
Maintenance dosage: 3 million IU three times/week.
For interferon alfa-2b
2 million IU/m² three times/week, subcutaneously or I.M.
Nursing considerations
- Make sure the patient's well-hydrated before and during treatment.
- Monitor him for flulike symptoms (fever, headache, fatigue, anorexia, nausea, and vomiting), which will probably abate as therapy progresses.
- To minimize flulike symptoms, give the drug at bedtime. Administer acetaminophen for fever and headache, as ordered.
- If the patient experiences severe adverse effects or the disease progresses rapidly, reduce doses 50%, withhold doses, or discontinue therapy, as ordered.
- If he will self-administer the drug at home, teach him the correct technique.
- Warn him against changing interferon brands, because recommended dosages differ.
- Instruct him to keep the drug in the refrigerator and to avoid freezing or shaking it.

Fine-needle biopsy: An alternative to surgery

In the past, a patient with a breast lump would probably need surgery for a definitive diagnosis. Today, she may have an alternative: fine-needle biopsy. Not only does this procedure spare her the trauma of surgery, but it also provides accurate diagnostic information fast; if necessary, she can begin appropriate therapy immediately. If the lump turns out to be a benign, fluid-filled cyst, the procedure eliminates the problem by aspirating the fluid.

Besides diagnosing breast lumps, fine-needle biopsy helps diagnose lesions in deep abdominal tissues, the lungs, the thyroid gland, salivary glands, lymph nodes, and skin. Contraindications include bleeding disorders and (for deep-tissue abdominal or thoracic biopsy) uncontrolled cough, severe pulmonary hypertension, and severe emphysema.

Because the patient doesn't need a general anesthetic, the doctor may perform a superficial-tissue biopsy in his office or in an outpatient clinic. (However, he may perform a deep-tissue biopsy in the hospital's radiology department so that he can use X-ray techniques for accurate needle placement.) By using a needle and syringe attached to a larger syringe pistol, he can manipulate the needle and syringe with one hand while steadying the tissue with the other. He'll advance the needle in short strokes to obtain specimens from several locations.

If you're assisting with the procedure:
- prepare the patient by explaining the procedure and describing the equipment. If she's undergoing a superficial-tissue biopsy, tell her she'll feel discomfort similar to what she'd feel during venipuncture. (If she's undergoing a deep-tissue biopsy, she'll receive a local anesthetic.)
- document baseline vital signs and make sure the patient has signed a consent form, if required.
- position her comfortably. Ask her to remain still during the procedure, but tell her to signal with her hand if she needs to cough or say something.
- remain with her and help her relax during the procedure.
- apply pressure to the site afterward, using a sterile gauze pad.
- tell her to report swelling, bleeding, or signs of infection.
- monitor for pneumothorax (following an upper chest biopsy).

The Ommaya reservoir: Providing access to CSF

Designed to deliver antibiotics, analgesics, and antineoplastic drugs to the CSF via the ventricles, the Ommaya reservoir spares a patient needing long-term therapy from repeated lumbar punctures. Besides providing convenient, comparatively painless access to CSF, it permits consistent and predictable drug distribution throughout the subarachnoid space and central nervous system. (Drugs given via lumbar puncture may escape into subdural or epidural spaces without ascending to the head.) As the Ommaya reservoir becomes more prevalent (some hospitals now use it to treat AIDS patients with CSF infections), you may soon care for a patient who has one.

Before reservoir insertion, the patient may receive either a local or general anesthetic, depending on his condition and the doctor's preference. Then the doctor drills a burr hole and inserts the device's catheter through the patient's nondominant frontal lobe into the lateral ventricle. The reservoir, which has a self-sealing silicone injection dome, rests over the burr hole under a scalp flap (see illustration). An X-ray confirms proper placement. Within 48 hours, the doctor can use the reservoir to deliver drugs, obtain CSF pressure measurements, drain CSF, and withdraw CSF specimens.

Nursing care
Before reservoir insertion, explain the procedure to your patient and answer his questions. Reassure him that his shaved hair will grow back—only a coin-sized patch must remain shaved for injections. Unless complications develop, his reservoir may function for years.

Provide incision care, as ordered. The doctor will probably leave a pressure dressing in place for 24 hours, then replace it with a gauze dressing. He'll remove the sutures in about 10 days. Instruct the patient to protect the site from bumps and trauma while he recovers.

If treated as an outpatient, the patient may resume normal activities within a short time, as directed. Tell him to notify the doctor if he experiences persistent headache, nausea, vomiting, or dizziness. *Note:* Under some circumstances, you may be responsible for teaching a family member how to administer drugs through the reservoir.

Complications
Teach your patient to report signs and symptoms of infection: headache, neck stiffness, and fever. The doctor can proba-bly treat an infection successfully by injecting antibiotics into the reservoir. Under some circumstances, however, he may remove the reservoir.

Another possible complication, catheter migration or blockage, sometimes—but not always—causes neurologic symptoms. If the doctor suspects such a problem, he may gently push and release the reservoir several times (a technique called pumping). Then, leaving his finger on the scalp, he feels for reservoir filling. Slow filling suggests catheter migration or blockage; a computed tomography scan confirms the diagnosis. The doctor corrects the problem surgically.

Note: If your patient's receiving antineoplastic drug therapy, monitor him closely for complications specific to the drug.

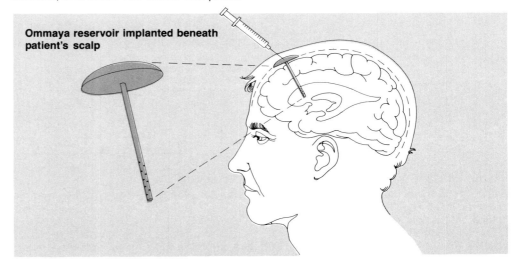

Ommaya reservoir implanted beneath patient's scalp

Preparing a patient for an Ommaya reservoir tap

• Describe the procedure to the patient and his family. Explain that his scalp over the reservoir will be shaved and an antimicrobial solution applied. The reservoir tap takes 15 to 30 minutes.
• Before prepping begins, make sure the patient isn't sensitive to iodine.
• Gather the equipment, as ordered. If the doctor will also inject a drug, obtain nonbacteriostatic sterile water, normal saline solution without preservative, or Elliott's B solution for drug dilution. *Important:* Use only 25G or smaller needles to puncture an Om-maya reservoir.
• Place the patient in Trendelenburg's position.
• During and after the procedure, monitor the patient for nausea and vomiting, headache, and dizziness.
• After the procedure, apply a sterile gauze square and apply gentle pressure for 1 to 2 minutes. The doctor will then apply a pressure bandage.
• Keep the patient flat, without a pillow, for 30 minutes, or as directed. Closely monitor his condition.

Diabetes

New methods and improved equipment help diabetic patients control their conditions and minimize long-term complications. In the following pages, we'll summarize the most recent developments in diabetes therapy and review current diabetes classifications. We'll also acquaint you with the Betatron II insulin pump, which enlists computer technology to help the patient maintain normal blood glucose levels.

UPDATE

Diabetes treatment: New therapies

Conventional diabetes therapy focuses on monitoring and controlling blood glucose levels. New therapies currently under development may further refine the process.

• **Pancreas islet cell grafts.** Grafted islet cells may help control blood glucose metabolism and prevent or resolve microangiopathic complications. However, this therapy requires pure, undamaged pancreas islet cells for grafting, and they're hard to obtain. Another obstacle: isolated islet cells are more likely to be rejected than islet-cell grafts in an intact pancreas.

• **Pancreas transplants.** Because of the high rejection risk, patients receiving pancreas transplants need immunosuppressive drug therapy. Unfortunately, long-term immunosuppression can cause more problems, including hepatotoxicity, nephrotoxicity, and infection. Consequently, most patients currently selected for pancreas transplantation are already receiving immunosuppressive agents for a previous transplant; they're also patients for whom diabetic complications pose a greater threat than long-term immunosuppression. A pancreas transplant may be performed by segmental pancreatic transplantation, pancreaticoduodenal transplantation, or simultaneous pancreatic transplantation.

• **Implantable probes and pumps.** Designed to monitor blood glucose levels and automatically deliver the correct insulin dose, implantable pumps offer the potential for more exact blood glucose control. However, problems with clogging and unreliable insulin secretion remain unresolved.

• **Cyclosporine therapy.** A promising treatment for Type I diabetes, cyclosporine therapy aims to prevent islet beta-cell destruction. Cyclosporine's immunosuppressive action may prevent circulating serum islet-cell antibodies from attacking islet cells.

• **Glycemic index.** This dietary therapy links blood glucose fluctuations with specific foods and identifies low-fat, starchy foods that diabetic patients can eat to increase carbohydrate intake without triggering high postprandial blood glucose levels. A patient must comply with therapy by determining his blood glucose level after every meal and snack.

Insulin infusion pumps: Key to better diabetes control

By delivering basal (small) insulin doses every few minutes and bolus doses at mealtimes, an insulin infusion pump helps a diabetic patient exert better control over his blood glucose levels. The CPI/Lilly Betatron II insulin pump featured on the following pages consists of a programmable microcomputer-based pump weighing less than 6 oz, an insulin reservoir, a rechargeable nickel cadmium battery pack, a backup lithium battery, and an infusion set. The patient inserts the needle at a subcutaneous injection site and carries the pump on his belt or in his pocket.

An insulin infusion pump offers several advantages over conventional insulin injection therapy. Small, frequent insulin doses released automatically, coupled with extra doses the patient releases at mealtimes, permit better blood glucose control—thus reducing long-term diabetic complications. Because the patient can adjust insulin dosage as circumstances warrant, he can be more flexible about what he eats and when he eats it.

The best candidates for insulin pump therapy include:

• people whose blood glucose levels fluctuate widely despite optimal insulin and dietary regimens

• people with variable work schedules or irregular mealtimes

• pregnant women, who may ensure a healthier pregnancy with more precise blood glucose control

• children or teenagers who aren't developing normally or who experience blood glucose fluctuations related to puberty.

As with self-injection therapy, insulin pump therapy requires the patient to know the basics of insulin pharmacology and blood glucose self-monitoring. He must also adhere to appropriate diet and exercise regimens. Consequently, the doctor probably won't order insulin pump therapy for:

• patients who won't or can't comply with standard dietary, insulin, and self-monitoring regimens

• those who miss medical appointments

• those who can't recognize hypoglycemia symptoms.

Patients with severe diabetic complications, such as advanced renal disease, proliferative retinopathy, or severe autonomic neuropathy, may also be poor candidates.

Programming the Betatron II insulin pump

If the doctor prescribes a Betatron II insulin infusion pump for your patient, teach him how to operate it. For example, help him learn to charge and insert the pump's batteries, as directed by the manufacturer.

Following the doctor's orders, the patient must also learn to program his pump to deliver a basal rate (the insulin amount released automatically over a 24-hour period) and bolus doses the patient gives himself before meals (if needed). Programmable functions include insulin concentration, basal rate, and meal (bolus) dose. However, the pump can perform six additional functions, including delivering an alternate basal rate and delaying a meal dose. In this photostory, we'll show you how to program concentration, basal rate, and meal dose; consult the manufacturer's manual for details on programming additional functions.

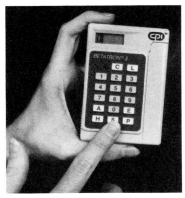

1 To program a value into one of the pump's functions, first call up the function by its assigned function code (see *Understanding Betatron II function codes* on page 56). To call up function codes 0 through 7, you'll press S (step), then the number corresponding to the function you want. *Caution:* Use your finger's side or pad to depress keys. A fingernail or other sharp object may damage the equipment.

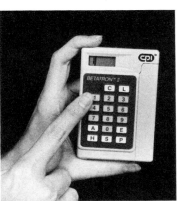

2 To program insulin concentration (U100 or U40), press S, then 1 (the function code for concentration). The digital display shows a 1 at its left end (see photo). *Note:* the right-hand portion may be blank, or it may display letters or digits.

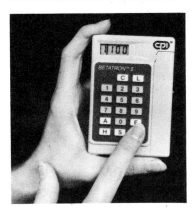

3 To program for U100, press 1,0,0; to program for U40, press 0,4,0. Then enter the concentration in the pump's microcomputer by pressing E (enter), as the nurse is doing here.

Note: Because you haven't yet entered a basal rate, your pump may now go to function 2 and sound an alarm. To stop the alarm, press C (clear); then proceed.

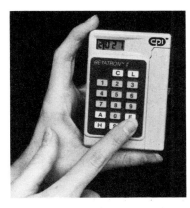

4 To program basal rate—the amount of insulin delivered daily, excluding meal doses and alternate basal infusions—call up the function by pressing S, then 2. If the doctor has prescribed 21 units of insulin per day, press 0,2,1, then E to enter the dose, as shown. (You can program any rate between 1 and 150 units.) *Note:* The patient can also program an alternate basal rate if the doctor recommends a different rate for a specified period.

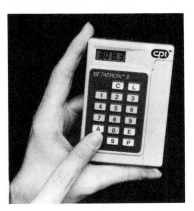

5 Now prepare to program the meal dose. If the patient's prescribed meal dose is 8.3 units, key in the appropriate numbers and press E. (Note the decimal point.)

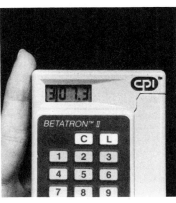

6 After entering the meal dose, the patient begins delivery by pressing A. (He can program the pump to deliver any meal dose between 0.1 and 20 units.) *Important:* The patient must clear and reprogram his meal dose whenever he changes insulin concentration.

7 As the pump delivers the dose, the display numbers count down (see photo) and the pump beeps as it delivers each unit. The patient can stop a meal dose during delivery simply by pressing C (clear). *Note:* The patient can preprogram meal doses for occasions when manual operation would be awkward—for example, when eating at a restaurant.

Diabetes

Preparing to use a Betatron II insulin pump

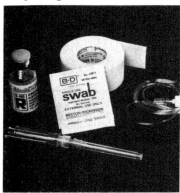

1 After teaching your patient to program his Betatron II pump, help him learn to set it up for use.

Besides the pump, obtain a vial of his prescribed insulin (at room temperature), an alcohol swab, a CPI/Lilly 9210 disposable reservoir, a CPI/Lilly infusion set, and tape or a bandage.

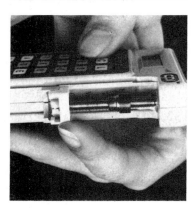

2 Slide the reservoir compartment cover off the pump. Release the locking cap from the drive nut by pulling the cap toward the reservoir scale's zero end, as the nurse has done here.

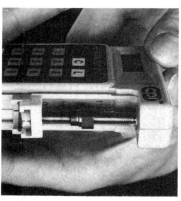

3 Determine the approximate amount of insulin needed by dividing the patient's daily dose (in units) by the insulin concentration. Then add the amount of insulin needed for priming (see chart on page 56). Line up the threads at the drive nut's front edge with the unit marking that corresponds to the insulin amount needed—in this case, 100 units.

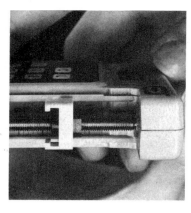

4 Fit the locking cap securely over the drive nut, as shown. Wipe the insulin vial's rubber diaphragm with the alcohol swab. Remove the reservoir from its wrapper.

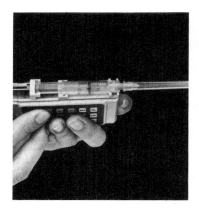

5 Place the reservoir into the reservoir compartment by positioning the plunger in the locking cap, as shown. Then snap the other end into place, as the nurse has done here. Make sure each end fits into its cradle and that the plunger rests firmly in the locking cap.

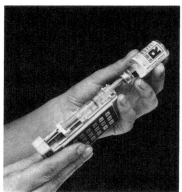

6 Remove the needle guard, invert the insulin vial, and pierce the vial's diaphragm with the needle.

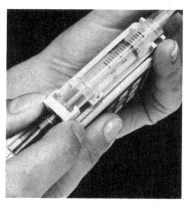

7 Then slide up the locking cap to force air out of the reservoir into the vial, as shown here.

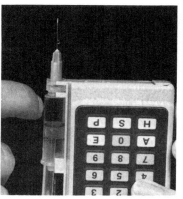

8 Draw insulin into the reservoir by sliding the locking cap down over the drive nut. Expel any air from the reservoir, as the nurse is doing here, using the same technique you'd use with an ordinary syringe. *Note:* Tell the patient to draw up only enough insulin for 1 day, to guard against accidental overdose.

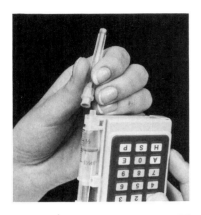

9 Replace the needle guard. Then unscrew the needle guard from the reservoir. Remove the needle and guard, as shown.

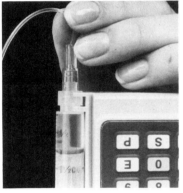

10 Now you're ready to connect the infusion set. Take the infusion set from its package and remove the sterile end cap from the Luer-Lok connector. Attach the infusion set to the reservoir with a gentle but firm twist. Replace the reservoir compartment cover.

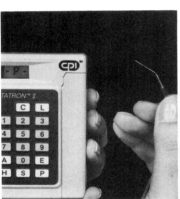

11 Use the pump's priming feature (function code 0) to prime the infusion set. Press S,0. Next, press and hold the P (prime) key until you see -P- in the display window (see photo) and you hear the pump beep. *Note:* If you decide against priming while the window displays -P-, just press C (clear).

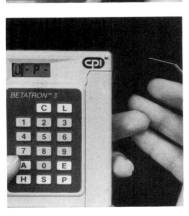

12 Then activate the priming feature by pressing and holding A (activate), as shown. Continue to hold A until insulin emerges from the needle and all air bubbles have been expelled. *Important:* Remind the patient to prime the pump whenever he disconnects the infusion set. If he replaces the reservoir but not the infusion set, he must prime the reservoir before reattaching the infusion set.

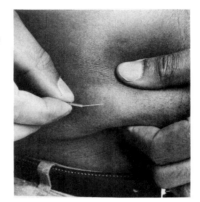

13 Now, after the patient has cleansed the insertion site, have him insert the needle at a subcutaneous site and secure it with a sterile dressing. Assess his technique and correct any problems. To reduce infection risk, the manufacturer recommends that the patient replace the infusion set and change the insertion site every 24 hours.

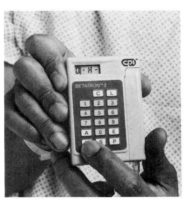

14 If the patient wants to disconnect the infusion set from the pump while the needle remains in place, he must first put the pump in hold by pressing S,0 and then pressing H until -H- appears in the display (see photo) and the pump beeps. (The pump beeps every 5 minutes that it's in hold.)

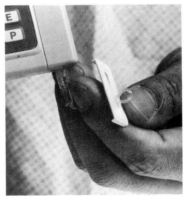

15 Next the patient should apply a slide clamp to guard against accidentally administering insulin. Instruct him to double the tubing before putting it into the clamp, as shown here, and to apply the clamp close to the pump.

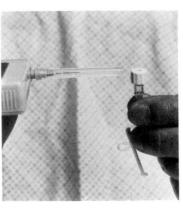

16 Disconnect the infusion set from the reservoir. Cap the infusion set and replace the needle (with needle guard in place) on the reservoir.
   Before reconnecting the infusion set, use the pump's prime feature to fill the infusion set's Luer-Lok connector with insulin. Reconnect the set and reservoir, and remove the slide clamp.

Diabetes

Understanding Betatron II function codes

Use these codes to program the Betatron II infusion pump (see the photostory on page 53).

Function	Description	Function code
Prime	Fills tubing with insulin	0
Hold	Stops insulin delivery	0
Delay-until-hold (automatic shutdown)	Monitors keyboard activity from 1 to 16 hours	0
Concentration	Adjusts dose based on insulin concentration (U40 or U100)	1
Basal rate	Infuses a programmed number of units of insulin over 24 hours	2
Meal dose	Delivers a programmed bolus insulin dose	3
Alternate basal rate	Enters an alternate basal rate	4
Alternate basal duration	Delivers the alternate basal rate for a determined length of time	5
Alternate basal delay	Delays the alternate basal rate delivery until after a number of minutes have elapsed	6
Accumulated dose	Shows total units of insulin received	7
Beeper control	Silences all beeps, except alarms	7
Reagent timer	Helps make blood and urine glucose measurements	7
Meal dose delay	Programs a delay before the meal dose is given	8
Dose limit	Programs a maximum insulin dose limit	9

How to determine priming volume

Use these guidelines to estimate the insulin volume you need to prime a Betatron II infusion set, as shown in the photostory beginning on page 54.

CPI infusion set	Priming volume
50 cm (20")	0.15 ml (15 units for U100; 6 units for U40)
100 cm (40")	0.25 ml (25 units for U100; 10 units for U40)
Extension	0.30 ml (30 units for U100; 12 units for U40)

Classifying glucose-intolerance disorders

The National Diabetes Data Group (NDDG) of the National Institutes of Health recognizes these categories of diabetes mellitus and other conditions related to glucose intolerance.

NDDG class	Former terms
Diabetes mellitus	
Type I. Insulin-dependent diabetes mellitus (IDDM)	• Juvenile diabetes, juvenile-onset diabetes, ketosis-prone diabetes, unstable or brittle diabetes
Type II. Non-insulin-dependent diabetes mellitus (NIDDM) • Nonobese NIDDM • Obese NIDDM (includes families with autosomal dominant inheritance)	• Adult-onset diabetes, maturity-onset diabetes, ketosis-resistant diabetes, stable diabetes
Other types, including diabetes mellitus associated with certain conditions and syndromes: pancreatic disease; hormonal, drug- or chemical-induced disorders; certain genetic syndromes; insulin receptor abnormalities	• Secondary diabetes
Impaired glucose tolerance (IGT)	
Nonobese IGT Obese IGT IGT associated with certain conditions and syndromes: pancreatic disease; hormonal, drug- or chemical-induced disorders; insulin receptor abnormalities; certain genetic syndromes	• Asymptomatic diabetes, chemical diabetes, latent diabetes, borderline diabetes, subclinical diabetes
Gestational diabetes	
Occurs only during pregnancy	• Gestational diabetes
Statistical risk classes	
Previous abnormality of glucose tolerance: patients now have normal glucose tolerance but previously had diabetic hyperglycemia or IGT, either spontaneously or in response to a known stimulus; includes former gestational and obese diabetics and others who have had transient hyperglycemia	• Subclinical diabetes, prediabetes, latent diabetes
Potential abnormality of glucose tolerance; includes persons who have never had abnormal glucose tolerance but who are at increased statistical risk for diabetes because of age, weight, race, or family history	• Prediabetes, potential diabetes

Diagnostic tests

Recent advances in medical technology have made magnetic resonance imaging (MRI) the diagnostic test of choice for certain disorders. Learn how to prepare a patient for MRI by reading the information at right.

In the following pages, you'll learn about two simple diagnostic tests you can do yourself. The Culturette Brand strep test identifies group A streptococcal bacteria directly from a throat swab, thus eliminating the time-consuming culture process. The Vacutainer Urine Collection Kit reduces the risk of false-positive culture results by providing a preservative for the specimen. For details, read on.

Using a Vacutainer Urine Collection Kit

How many times have you sent a urine specimen to the lab for culture and later found yourself asking the patient for another specimen because contaminant overgrowth caused a false-positive result? A new Vacutainer product designed to prevent contaminant overgrowth could save you—and your patients—needless frustration.

The Vacutainer Urine Collection Kit consists of a collection cup, a lid with transfer device, a Vacutainer tube with preservative, and two patient cleansing wipes. The system allows you to collect specimens for culture and urinalysis without pouring urine from cup to tube. Just transfer urine from the collection cup to the Vacutainer tube, using the simple, spillproof procedure shown in this photostory. The tube's preservative prevents bacteria from multiplying for at least 24 hours—without refrigeration.

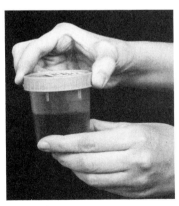

1 Teach the patient how to collect a clean-catch, midstream urine specimen and give him the collection kit. Warn him against touching the inside of the cup or the underside of the lid (including the straw-shaped structure). Also tell him not to remove the paper label on the lid's top.

When he returns with the specimen, make sure he screwed the lid on the cup securely.

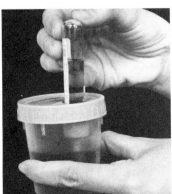

2 Then peel back the protective paper label, and push the tube into the lid's recessed channel. Urine will immediately flow into the tube. Hold the tube in place until the flow stops. *Note:* Perform this step within 20 minutes of urine collection.

Remove the tube and shake it to dissolve the preservative. Replace the paper label on the lid. Label both tube and cup, and send them to the laboratory.

UPDATE

Learning about magnetic resonance imaging

Similar to computed tomography (CT), magnetic resonance imaging (MRI) produces cross-sectional tissue images in multiple planes. Unlike CT, however, MRI relies on radio frequency waves to generate images. During MRI scanning, the patient lies within a magnetic field and radio waves stimulate selected portions of his body. The MRI computer produces images based on energy changes in each section. (In CT scanning, the image reflects tissue density differences detected on X-ray.) MRI's superior soft tissue contrasts provide a clear view of blood vessels and permit differentiation of healthy, benign, and malignant tissues.

Entirely safe and noninvasive, MRI eliminates risks associated with the X-rays and iodine-based contrast media needed for CT.

Disadvantages and drawbacks

While superior in many ways to CT, MRI has a few disadvantages. For example, the patient must lie still longer—for 5- to 20-minute intervals—during the procedure, which may last up to 90 minutes. The quicker CT procedure may be a better choice for children and for adults with back or breathing problems. Other patients who shouldn't undergo MRI include:

• those with certain implants, including metallic vascular clips for cerebral aneurysms, metal-containing heart valves (the magnetic force may dislodge metal objects), implanted insulin pumps or transcutaneous electrical nerve stimulation devices, and pacemakers (the magnetic field could cause pacemaker malfunction). Patients with shrapnel should also forgo MRI. *Note:* Some metal objects safely withstand MRI—for example, hip prostheses, intrauterine devices, dental fillings and braces, sternal wire sutures, ear endoprostheses, and tantalum mesh.

• obese patients who may not fit in the magnetic tunnel

• pregnant women, because MRI's effects on a fetus remain unknown

• unstable patients and those needing life-support equipment. Most supportive equipment, including oxygen tanks, defibrillators, and I.V. infusion pumps, can't be used during MRI.

Nursing considerations

A patient undergoing an abdominal scan can't have anything by mouth for 4 to 6 hours beforehand. But most other patients won't have any pre-test restrictions. Suggest that your patient use the bathroom before the test begins.

Tell him to remove all metal items before leaving his room. (He'll be checked again at the scanner room door.) Also tell him to leave behind any cards with metallic strips (such as bank or credit cards)—the scanner could erase them.

Equally important, tell the patient what to expect. Without proper preparation, he may become claustrophobic in the scanner tunnel. Don't forget to cover these points:

• During the procedure, he'll lie on a narrow stretcher that fits in the tunnel. Assure him that he'll be constantly monitored throughout the procedure.

• He won't feel anything (including pain) from MRI. However, he may become uncomfortable lying on the narrow stretcher for an hour or more. But mirrors at his head and an intercom (or call button) should lessen feelings of claustrophobia, and fans keep air circulating in the tunnel.

• The machine makes thumping noises during the procedure. He may want to wear earplugs.

Diagnostic tests

Using Culturette Brand 10-Minute Group A Strep ID

Group A streptococci cause more tonsil and pharyngeal infections than any other bacterial strain. Treated promptly, these strep infections respond quickly to antibiotic therapy. Left untreated, they can cause serious complications, such as rheumatic fever and glomerulonephritis.

Until recently, positive diagnosis depended on throat cultures. Unfortunately, culture results may not be available for 2 days, which delays antibiotic therapy for some patients without classic strep throat symptoms. Another drawback: accurate interpretation requires training and skill.

A recently developed alternative to throat cultures, the highly accurate Culturette Brand 10-Minute Group A Strep ID detects group A strep antigens collected on throat swabs. You can perform the test and interpret results in minutes, while the patient waits. This photostory shows you how.

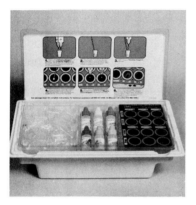

1 The Culturette kit contains a positive and a negative reagent, three extraction reagents, a detection reagent, microtubes, micropipettes, test slides, and sterile swabs. Set up one microtube for each specimen and number them appropriately.

Using a sterile swab, obtain a throat specimen (see the box on the following page).

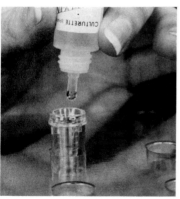

2 Place one drop of Extraction Reagent 1 into the microtube. Then add one drop of Extraction Reagent 2.

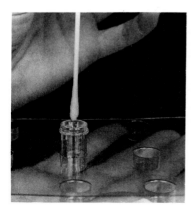

3 Place the swab into the microtube, as shown, and mix well. Leave the swab in the solution for at least 5 minutes (at room temperature).

Next, add two drops of Extraction Reagent 3. Roll the swab against the microtube walls; then briefly leave it in the solution for maximum absorption.

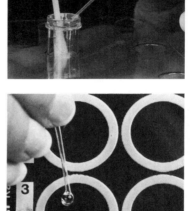

4 Squeeze a micropipette's bulb to expel air. Then, press the swab against the microtube's bottom. Insert the micropipette's tip into the bottom of the microtube, and extract a fluid specimen directly from the swab.

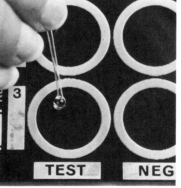

5 Place one drop on the *test* circle and one on the *negative* circle. Then, gently agitate the Negative Control Reagent and Detection Reagent 4 bottles. Add one free-falling drop of Negative Control Reagent to the *negative* circle and one free-falling drop of Detection Reagent 4 to the *test* circle. Hold the reagent bottles upright to ensure proper drop delivery.

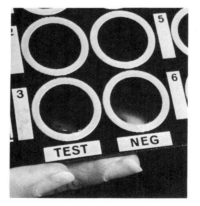

6 Mix the liquids in each circle with a clean applicator stick. Then, hold the slide plate under a strong incandescent light and gently rock it at a 45-degree angle in each direction. (Or use a mechanical rotator set at 90 to 140 rpm.)

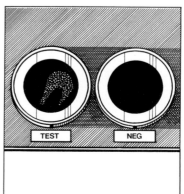

7 While rocking the plate, watch closely for signs of agglutination. Any amount of agglutination in the *test* circle that's greater than that in the *negative* circle indicates a positive test result (see illustration). A homogenous milky appearance indicates a negative result. *Important:* Interpret results immediately. After 3 minutes, drying may make results inaccurate.

Strep testing: Special considerations

To assure accuracy when using the Culturette Brand 10-minute Group A Strep ID, follow the manufacturer's recommendations, which include the following:
• Wash and dry the slide plate before and after use, according to the manufacturer's instructions.
• Perform a positive control test when first using a new kit and periodically thereafter (according to hospital or laboratory protocol). Add one drop each of Extraction Reagents 1 and 2 to a microtube; then add two drops of Positive Control Reagent. Place an applicator stick (instead of a swab) in the microtube and continue the procedure, as shown in the preceding photostory. You should see strong to moderate agglutination in the *test* circle and no agglutination in the *negative* circle. Don't use the reagents if you see no reaction or only a weak reaction in the *test* circle.
• Use proper technique to obtain a throat specimen. First, depress the tongue and expose the throat. With the throat well illuminated, firmly rub a sterile swab over the posterior pharynx, including the tonsils or tonsillar fossae and any inflamed areas. Don't let the swab touch the tongue, lips, or cheeks.
• Allow reagents to warm to room temperature before using. Before opening dropper bottles, tap the bottoms on a table to drive the liquid to the bottom.
• Gently invert the latex suspensions (Detection Reagent 4 and Negative Control Reagent) before use to resuspend latex beads.
• If test results aren't consistent with the patient's signs and symptoms, obtain a specimen for a follow-up throat culture.

SI units: A change in diagnostic documentation

A revolution in clinical laboratory measurement has begun: soon, most laboratory values will be recorded according to the International System of Units (SI units). This means that you'll be working with test results expressed in unfamiliar units of measurement. By starting to learn about SI units now, you minimize the risk of misinterpreting laboratory results later.

Widely used outside the United States, SI units grew out of the metric system. They provide a coherent value system that permits easier comparison of values for different properties.

You're already familiar with some SI units, such as the kilogram. But in American laboratories, most common chemical and hematologic values have always been reported in other units of measurement. By adopting SI units, American professionals improve their ability to interpret biological relationships and their ability to communicate with the international medical community.

The Medical and Health Coordinating Group of the American National Metric Council initiated the change to SI units. To minimize errors, the group advocates a gradual conversion. The American Medical Association (AMA), among other professional organizations, endorses this recommendation.

In July 1986, AMA journals began providing SI unit measurements after conventional laboratory values. By July 1988, these journals will provide laboratory values in SI units only.

Among other things, the change to SI units means that you must learn new "panic values" for most measurements you routinely rely upon. An exception: blood pressure measurements, which you'll continue to express in millimeters of mercury—not in kilopascals, the equivalent SI unit.

Classifying SI units

SI units fall into three categories: *base units,* such as the meter and the kilogram; *derived base units,* such as the cubic meter; and *supplementary units,* such as the radian and the steradian. The following examples show how a few common hematology and blood chemistry values will be expressed in SI units.

Substance	Current reference intervals (examples)	Present unit	SI unit reference intervals	SI unit symbol
Glucose (fasting)	70-110	mg/dl	3.9-6.1	mmol/l
Hematocrit (female)	33-43	%	0.33-0.43	1
Hemoglobin (female)	12.0-15.0	g/dl	120-150	g/l
Platelet count	130-400	10^3 or mm^3	130-400	10^9/l
Potassium	3.5-5.0	mEq/l or mg/dl	3.5-5.0	mmol/l

Adapted from *Annals of Internal Medicine,* vol. 106, no. 1, 118-29.

Drug therapy

Every year the Food and Drug Administration approves many new drugs. In the following pages, we'll introduce you to a few of the recently approved drugs you may administer to medical/surgical patients, including:
• buspirone for treating anxiety
• norfloxacin for treating certain urinary tract infections
• famotidine for treating duodenal ulcers
• buprenorphine for pain relief.

As always, thoroughly familiarize yourself with any drug before administering it. Use the chart on pages 62 to 64 as a guide, but consult package inserts for complete information.

Read these two pages for details on monoclonal antibodies, which may contribute to new drug therapies in the future, and for the latest adult vaccination guidelines.

Monoclonal antibodies: Magic bullets?

Called "magic bullets" by some, monoclonal antibodies might be better termed "guided missiles" for their ability to recognize and target specific antigens, including tumor cells, microorganisms, and hormones. The new drug muromonab-CD3 (see page 63) uses a monoclonal antibody to attack cells responsible for kidney transplant rejection.

To produce monoclonal antibodies, researchers inject a mouse with the target antigen, stimulating it to produce specific antibodies. They then remove these antibodies from the mouse's spleen and fuse them with myeloma cells taken from another mouse. When injected into a mouse, the resulting cells (hybridomas) have a virtually unlimited ability to reproduce the desired antibody.

Research and diagnosis

Although still in its infancy, monoclonal antibody therapy already has a place in medical research and diagnostic testing.

Coupling monoclonal antibodies with radioactive tags permits researchers to learn more about such disorders as Type I insulin-dependent diabetes mellitus and kidney disease. Diagnostic tests employing monoclonal antibodies can identify sexually transmitted diseases and detect tumors so small that they'd escape detection by other tests. Similarly, specially programmed antibodies can highlight damaged heart tissue. Home ovulation and pregnancy tests also use monoclonal antibodies.

Treatment

Currently used to fight transplant rejection, monoclonal antibodies may soon have other therapeutic uses. For example, they may someday help the body resist autoimmune disorders. And they could also play an important role in cancer therapy by carrying antineoplastic chemicals to cancer cells without disturbing surrounding healthy tissue.

Monoclonal antibody formation

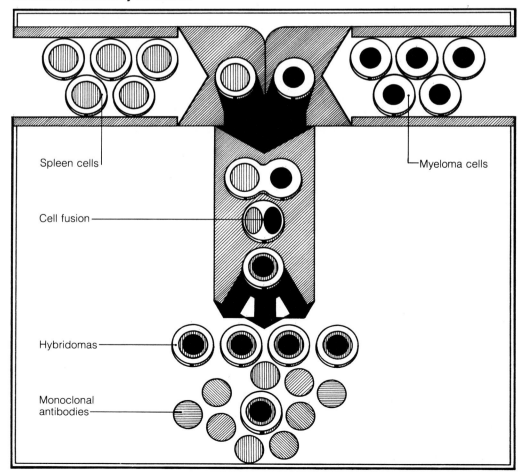

Spleen cells

Myeloma cells

Cell fusion

Hybridomas

Monoclonal antibodies

Adult vaccination: New recommendations

Recently, the Centers for Disease Control and the American College of Physicians published guidelines for routine immunization of adults living in the United States. These guidelines recommend the following six vaccinations for routine use. According to the guidelines, the vaccines for influenza, pneumococcus, and hepatitis B should be used more widely than they are at present.

Vaccine	Indications/Dosage	Possible adverse effects	Nursing considerations
Hepatitis B—chemically inactivated hepatitis B surface antigen (HBsAg) particles	For all high-risk people—male homosexuals, intravenous drug abusers, people who have household or sexual contacts with hepatitis B carriers, dialysis patients, people receiving clotting Factors VIII or XI, mortuary workers, medical or laboratory workers frequently exposed to blood or blood products, and residents and staff of institutions for the mentally retarded: three doses (each 1 ml I.M. in the deltoid muscle), with the second dose given after 1 month, the third after 6 months; double doses for immunocompromised patients	Local pain	• Hepatitis B vaccination doesn't predispose recipients to acquired immune deficiency syndrome (AIDS); in fact, the human immunodeficiency virus, which causes AIDS, is inactivated during preparation of the hepatitis B vaccine. • Infants born to mothers who test positive for HBsAg should receive both the vaccine and hepatitis B immune globulin. • Pregnancy isn't a contraindication; the vaccine poses no risk to the fetus, and hepatitis B infection in a pregnant woman can cause problems for the mother and fetus.
Influenza—inactivated whole virus or subunits grown in chick embryo cells	For all high-risk people—patients with diabetes or other metabolic diseases, severe anemia, or chronic pulmonary, cardiovascular, or renal disease; immunosuppressed patients; patients in chronic care facilities; all people over age 65; and health care professionals who have contact with high-risk people: one dose (0.5 ml I.M.) annually	Fever, chills, myalgia, malaise	• Influenza vaccination is contraindicated in people who are allergic to eggs. • Whole virus vaccine is contraindicated in children under age 13. • Adverse reactions occur only rarely. • Influenza and pneumococcal vaccinations can be given concomitantly at different sites safely and effectively.
Measles—attenuated live virus grown in chick fibroblasts*	A single dose (0.5 ml S.C.) of live measles vaccine for every person born after 1956 who didn't receive live measles vaccine after age 1 and who doesn't have absolute proof of immunity (a documented history of measles infection or laboratory evidence of immunity) A single dose of live vaccine for all people vaccinated between 1963 and 1967 with inactivated measles vaccine, to prevent severe atypical measles	Low-grade fever	• Live measles vaccination is contraindicated in people who are allergic to eggs; those who have experienced a hypersensitivity reaction to neomycin; pregnant women; and immunocompromised patients. • People born in or before 1956 are probably immune to measles. • About 1 in 10 people develops mild symptoms of attenuated measles (fever, malaise, anorexia, characteristic rash) 5 to 10 days after vaccination.
Pneumococcal—polysaccharides from 23 types of *Streptococcus pneumoniae*	For all high-risk people—patients with chronic cardiac or pulmonary disease, alcoholism, cirrhosis, diabetes, Hodgkin's disease, nephrotic syndrome, renal failure, cerebrospinal fluid leaks, immunosuppression, and other conditions that predispose to pneumococcal infection (particularly asplenism and sickle-cell anemia); and all people over age 65: one dose (0.5 ml S.C. or I.M.)	Local pain and erythema	• Pneumococcal vaccine is effective for most people with normal immune function, but not for severely immunocompromised patients. • Vaccination is contraindicated in previously immunized people, even those who received an older vaccine that contained fewer pneumococcal types. • Pneumococcal and influenza vaccinations may be given concomitantly at different sites.
Rubella—attenuated live virus grown in human diploid cells (RA 27/3 strain)*	One dose (0.5 ml S.C.) for all unimmunized women of childbearing age and all pediatric or obstetric care workers who don't have laboratory evidence of immunity	Low-grade fever, rash, lymphadenopathy, sore throat, arthralgias, and arthritis	• Contraindicated in pregnant women, people with hypersensitivity to neomycin, and immunocompromised patients. • About 40% of people receiving the vaccine develop joint pain after vaccination; frank arthritis is rare.
Tetanus-diphtheria (Adult Td)—adsorbed tetanus and diphtheria toxoids	A primary series of immunizations (two doses of 0.5 ml I.M., given 1 to 2 months apart; then one dose 6 months later) for all unimmunized people One Td booster injection every 10 years for everyone	Local pain and swelling	• Contraindicated in anyone who had a hypersensitivity reaction to a previous dose. • Severe local pain and swelling can result from too-frequent Td booster injections. • Pertussis vaccine (combined with diphtheria and tetanus toxoids for children) isn't recommended for adults.

*May be given as combined measles-rubella or measles-mumps-rubella vaccine.

Drug therapy

Drug update
Follow these dosage guidelines for adult patients. Consult package inserts for more detailed information.

Betaxolol (Betoptic)

Ophthalmic beta-adrenergic blocker

Indications
● Chronic open-angle glaucoma
● Ocular hypertension

Dosage
One drop twice a day

Nursing considerations
● Tell the patient that his eye may sting and tear briefly after drug instillation.
● Closely monitor diabetic patients; the drug may mask signs of acute hypoglycemia. Also monitor patients taking oral beta blockers (watch for additive drug effects) and those taking reserpine (watch for hypotension and bradycardia).
● Although uncommon, such systemic reactions as insomnia and depressive neurosis develop in some patients.

Bitolterol (Tornalate)

Orally inhaled bronchodilator

Indications
● Bronchial asthma
● Reversible bronchospasm

Dosage
To treat bronchospasm, two inhalations 1 to 3 minutes apart, followed by a third inhalation, if needed. To prevent bronchospasm, two inhalations every 8 hours. (Dosage shouldn't exceed three inhalations every 6 hours or two inhalations every 4 hours.)

Nursing considerations
● Teach the patient how to use his inhaler.
● Monitor respiratory function and watch for adverse effects: tremors, nervousness, headache, dizziness, palpitations, chest discomfort, tachycardia, coughing, and throat irritation.
● Tell the patient that adverse effects should disappear within an hour after drug administration. Instruct him to report severe or prolonged reactions.

Buprenorphine (Buprenex)

Opioid analgesic (Schedule V controlled substance); also has a narcotic-antagonist action

Indication
● Moderate to severe pain

Dosage
0.3 mg I.M. or slow I.V. injection at 6-hour intervals around the clock or p.r.n. Maximum per dose: 0.6 mg.

Nursing considerations
● Observe the patient for adverse reactions: sedation, nausea, dizziness, headache, vomiting, miosis, sweating, hypotension, and hypoventilation.
● Closely monitor the patient if he's receiving another drug that affects central nervous system (CNS) function; buprenorphine increases CNS effects.
● Also monitor a patient with compromised respiratory function; buprenorphine may decrease respiratory rate or cause severe respiratory depression. (Naloxone [Narcan] won't completely reverse respiratory depression caused by buprenorphine.)
● Don't give the drug to a narcotic-dependent patient; it may precipitate withdrawal symptoms.

Buspirone (BuSpar)

Antianxiety drug

Indications
● Anxiety disorders
● Short-term anxiety

Dosage
5 mg three times a day initially; increase dosage 5 mg/day at 2- to 3-day intervals, as needed. Maximum daily dose: 60 mg.

Nursing considerations
● Buspirone has no sedative effects and won't potentiate alcohol; however, it may make the patient feel restless.
● The drug may not produce full therapeutic effects for 1 to 2 weeks.
● A patient who previously took a benzodiazepine drug may be less responsive to buspirone than other patients.
● Although sedative effects are unlikely, warn the patient against driving and other activities requiring alertness until he determines how the drug affects him.

Ceftazidime (Fortaz, Tazicef, Tazidime)

Third-generation cephalosporin

Indications
● Infection of the lower respiratory tract, lower urinary tract, skin, abdomen, bones, joints, CNS, or reproductive organs by susceptible organisms, notably *Pseudomonas aeruginosa*
● Septicemia caused by susceptible organisms
● Respiratory tract infection in patients with cystic fibrosis

Dosage
1 g I.M. or I.V. every 8 to 12 hours. Maximum daily dose: 6 g.

Nursing considerations
● Before reconstituting the drug, read the package insert carefully.
● Monitor the patient for adverse effects: pruritus, fever, rash, diarrhea, eosinophilia, thrombocytosis, positive Coombs' test without hemolysis, elevated hepatic enzyme levels, phlebitis, and inflammation at injection site.

Enalapril (Vasotec)

Antihypertensive drug

Indication
● Hypertension

Dosage
5 mg P.O. once a day initially; then adjust according to response. Usual dosage range: 10 to 40 mg daily as a single dose or in two divided doses.

Nursing considerations
● As ordered, instruct the patient to discontinue diuretic therapy before beginning enalapril therapy, to reduce the risk of hypotension. (Diuretic therapy may be reinstated later, if necessary.)
● Observe the patient for angioedema (including laryngeal edema), especially after the first dose. Instruct him to report breathing difficulty and swelling in his face, eyes, lips, or tongue.
● Monitor for other adverse effects, including hypotension, headache, dizziness, and fatigue.
● Tell the patient to report fever, sore throat, and other signs of infection. Rarely, the drug may cause neutropenia or agranulocytosis, making him susceptible to infection.

Etretinate (Tegison)

Systemic antipsoriatic drug

Indication
● Severe psoriasis unresponsive to standard therapy

Dosage
To achieve initial response, give 0.75 to 1 mg/kg/day in divided doses for 8 to 16 weeks. (Erythrodermic psoriasis may respond to a lower initial dosage of 0.25 mg/kg/day; as needed, the daily dosage may be increased by 0.25 mg/kg at weekly intervals. Maximum dosage: 1.5 mg/kg/day.)
   After initial response, give maintenance doses of 0.5 to 0.75 mg/kg/day.

Nursing considerations
● Contraindicated for pregnant women, for fertile women who wish to become pregnant, and for fertile women who don't practice effective birth control: etretinate causes major fetal abnormalities.
● Tell a female patient that she must avoid becoming pregnant before, during, and after therapy (for an indefinite period).
● Monitor the patient for adverse effects: thirst, mouth soreness, hair loss, dry skin, itching, bone or joint pain, fatigue, eye irritation, and abdominal pain.
● Instruct the patient to take the drug with food.
● Tell him to avoid vitamin A supplements, which may contribute to additive toxic effects.
● Warn him that his psoriasis may flare up temporarily after he begins therapy.
● If he wears contact lenses, tell him that the drug may diminish his tolerance for them.

Famotidine (Pepcid)

Histamine (H$_2$) blocker

Indications
- Active duodenal ulcer (short-term therapy)
- Healed duodenal ulcer (maintenance therapy)
- Pathological hypersecretory conditions—for example, Zollinger-Ellison syndrome and multiple endocrine adenomas

Dosage
For duodenal ulcer
Acute therapy: 40 mg once a day at bedtime or 20 mg b.i.d.
Maintenance therapy: 20 mg once a day at bedtime.
For pathological hypersecretory conditions
Variable according to patient's condition. A typical patient may receive 20 mg every 6 hours; however, a few patients need as much as 160 mg every 6 hours.

Nursing considerations
- Most patients treated for active duodenal ulcers respond within 4 weeks; acute therapy rarely continues longer than 8 weeks.
- A patient receiving famotidine for hypersecretory conditions may continue therapy for as long as clinically indicated.
- The patient may take antacids concomitantly, as ordered.
- If he's taking one daily dose, remind him to take it at bedtime.

Imipenem/Cilastatin sodium (Primaxin)

Broad-spectrum antibiotic (imipenem) combined with an enzyme inhibitor (cilastatin); cilastatin slows renal metabolism of imipenem and permits it to treat urinary tract infection

Indications
- Infection of lower respiratory tract, lower urinary tract skin, abdomen, reproductive organs, bones, and joints by susceptible organisms (most gram-positive and gram-negative bacteria)
- Septicemia
- Endocarditis

Dosage
250 mg to 1 g I.V. every 6 to 8 hours, not to exceed 50 mg/kg or 4 g daily (whichever is less). Infuse 250- and 500-mg doses over 20 to 30 minutes; 1-g doses over 40 to 60 minutes.

Nursing considerations
- Imipenem treats many infections that otherwise would require therapy with a combination of antibiotics. Unlike aminoglycosides, imipenem isn't ototoxic or nephrotoxic.
- Imipenem/cilastatin has a short duration of action, so you may give it more frequently than other antibiotics.
- Keep the patient well hydrated during therapy.
- If he becomes nauseated, slow the infusion rate.

- Monitor him for other adverse effects: phlebitis, pain at injection site, vomiting, diarrhea, rash, fever, and CNS symptoms (myoclonic activity, confusion, or seizures).

Midazolam (Versed)

Sedative and amnesic (Schedule IV controlled substance)

Indications
- Preoperative sedation
- Induction of general anesthesia

Dosage
To sedate and relieve anxiety preoperatively
0.07 to 0.08 mg/kg I.M. about 1 hour before surgery (may be given with atropine or scopolamine and with reduced narcotics doses)
To produce conscious sedation before short procedures
0.1 to 0.15 mg/kg by slow I.V. injection immediately before the procedure. Give up to 0.2 mg/kg if the patient isn't also receiving narcotics.
To induce general anesthesia
0.3 to 0.35 mg/kg I.V. over 20 to 30 seconds. As needed, give additional increments (25% of the initial dose) to complete induction. Maximum total dose: 0.6 mg/kg.

Nursing considerations
- Have oxygen and resuscitation equipment nearby before beginning the infusion; midazolam can cause severe respiratory depression.
- As ordered, you may mix midazolam in the same syringe with morphine, meperidine, atropine, or scopolamine.
- For I.M. administration, inject deeply into a large muscle mass.
- For I.V. administration, take care to avoid extravasation.
- Monitor the patient for variations in blood pressure and pulse rate, especially if he was premedicated with a narcotic. Other possible adverse effects include headache, oversedation, nausea and vomiting, hiccups, and pain at the injection site.

Monooctanoin (Moctanin)

Gallstone-solubilizing drug

Indication
- Cholesterol gallstones

Dosage
3 to 5 ml/hour, perfused at a pressure of 10 cmH$_2$0 for 7 to 21 days

Nursing considerations
- Before beginning the infusion, warm monooctanoin to 60° to 80° F. (15.6° to 26.7° C.). During the infusion, don't let its temperature fall below 65° F. (18.4° C.).
- Continuously perfuse the drug through a catheter inserted directly into the common bile duct.
- Regulate the infusion with a peristaltic infusion pump to ensure that perfusion pressure doesn't exceed 15 cmH$_2$0. (An outpatient can use a portable pump with a pressure safety device.)

- Discontinue the infusion when the patient eats, to minimize gastrointestinal (GI) irritation.
- Monitor for adverse GI effects: pain, nausea, vomiting, and diarrhea.
- Monitor GI function for signs of gallbladder or liver dysfunction. The doctor will order routine liver function tests during therapy, to check for metabolic acidosis.
- As ordered, discontinue therapy after 10 days if endoscopy or X-rays reveal that stones haven't been dissolved or reduced in size.

Muromonab-CD3 (Orthoclone OKT3)

Monoclonal antibody for treating allograft rejection

Indication
- Acute allograft rejection in renal transplant patients

Dosage
5 mg I.V. bolus once a day for 10 to 14 days

Nursing considerations
- As ordered, reduce concomitant immunosuppressive therapy during muromonab-CD3 therapy; also reduce or discontinue cyclosporine. Resume maintenance immunosuppression about 3 days before the end of muromonab-CD3 therapy.
- Carefully assess the patient before beginning therapy. Notify the doctor if the patient has a fever (temperature shouldn't exceed 100° F. [37.8° C.] before the first dose) or if you see signs of fluid overload. A patient with fluid overload before treatment may develop severe pulmonary edema. *Important:* Be prepared to administer cardiopulmonary resuscitation if the patient develops complications during therapy.
- As ordered, give methylprednisolone sodium succinate 1 mg/kg I.V. before muromonab-CD3 administration and hydrocortisone sodium succinate 100 mg I.V. 30 minutes afterward. These drugs help minimize adverse effects following the first dose (fever, chills, dyspnea, and malaise). The doctor may also order concomitant doses of acetaminophen and antihistamines.
- Draw up muromonab-CD3 into a syringe through a low protein-binding 0.2 or 0.22 micrometer filter. Discard the filter and attach the needle. Administer the bolus injection in less than 1 minute. (You may see fine, translucent particles in the drug; these don't affect its potency.) *Caution:* Don't give muromonab-CD3 by I.V. infusion or mix it with other drugs.
- Inform the patient about possible adverse effects and tell him that they will probably lessen as therapy progresses.
- Closely monitor him for 48 hours after the first dose.
- Store the drug in the refrigerator. Don't freeze or shake it.

Drug therapy

Drug update continued

Norfloxacin (Noroxin)

Broad-spectrum antibacterial drug

Indication
• Urinary tract infection by susceptible organisms, including *Escherichia coli, Klebsiella pneumoniae, Proteus mirabilis, Pseudomonas aeruginosa, Staphylococcus aureus,* and group D streptococci

Dosage
400 mg twice daily for 7 to 10 days for uncomplicated urinary tract infection; 400 mg twice daily for 10 to 21 days for complicated urinary tract infection. Maximum daily dose: 800 mg.

Nursing considerations
• Contraindicated for children and pregnant women.
• Make sure the patient's well hydrated before therapy begins. Instruct him to drink plenty of fluids throughout therapy to maintain good urinary output and prevent crystalluria.
• Tell him to take each dose with a glass of water, either 1 hour before or 2 hours after a meal.
• Tell him to avoid taking antacids for 2 hours after taking a norfloxacin dose.

• Inform him that the drug may cause dizziness. Advise him to avoid driving and other activities requiring alertness until he determines how the drug affects him.

Suprofen (Suprol)

Nonsteroidal anti-inflammatory drug

Indications
• Mild to moderate pain
• Primary dysmenorrhea
Note: Because of possible adverse renal effects, other drugs should be tried first.

Dosage
200 mg every 4 to 6 hours as needed. Maximum daily dose: 800 mg.

Nursing considerations
• Contraindicated for patients hypersensitive to aspirin or other nonsteroidal anti-inflammatory drugs.
• Tell him to report adverse effects, which may include flank pain, GI symptoms (nausea, dyspepsia, diarrhea, constipation, or bleeding), vision disturbances, skin rash, weight gain, and edema. The doctor will discontinue the drug if the patient develops nephrotoxicity, blood dyscrasias, or other severe adverse effects.

• Advise the patient to take suprofen on an empty stomach, if possible. If the drug causes GI upset, however, he may take it with a little milk or an antacid.
• Tell him to use the drug only as directed—it's not recommended for long-term use.

Terfenadine (Seldane)

Antihistamine

Indication
• Seasonal allergic rhinitis (hay fever)

Dosage
60 mg twice a day

Nursing considerations
• Contraindicated for children under age 12.
• Tell the patient he may experience a dry mouth and throat. Unlike most antihistamines, however, terfenadine doesn't cause drowsiness and it seems less likely to cause anticholinergic reactions.
• Advise the patient to check the drug label carefully—in several cases, terfenadine (Seldane) prescriptions have been mistakenly filled with piroxicam (Feldene).

A new look for some familiar drugs

As a nurse, you must be familiar with a drug's shape and markings. The chart below illustrates recent changes in some drug shapes and/or markings. In each example, the upper illustration represents the old look; the lower illustration, the new look.

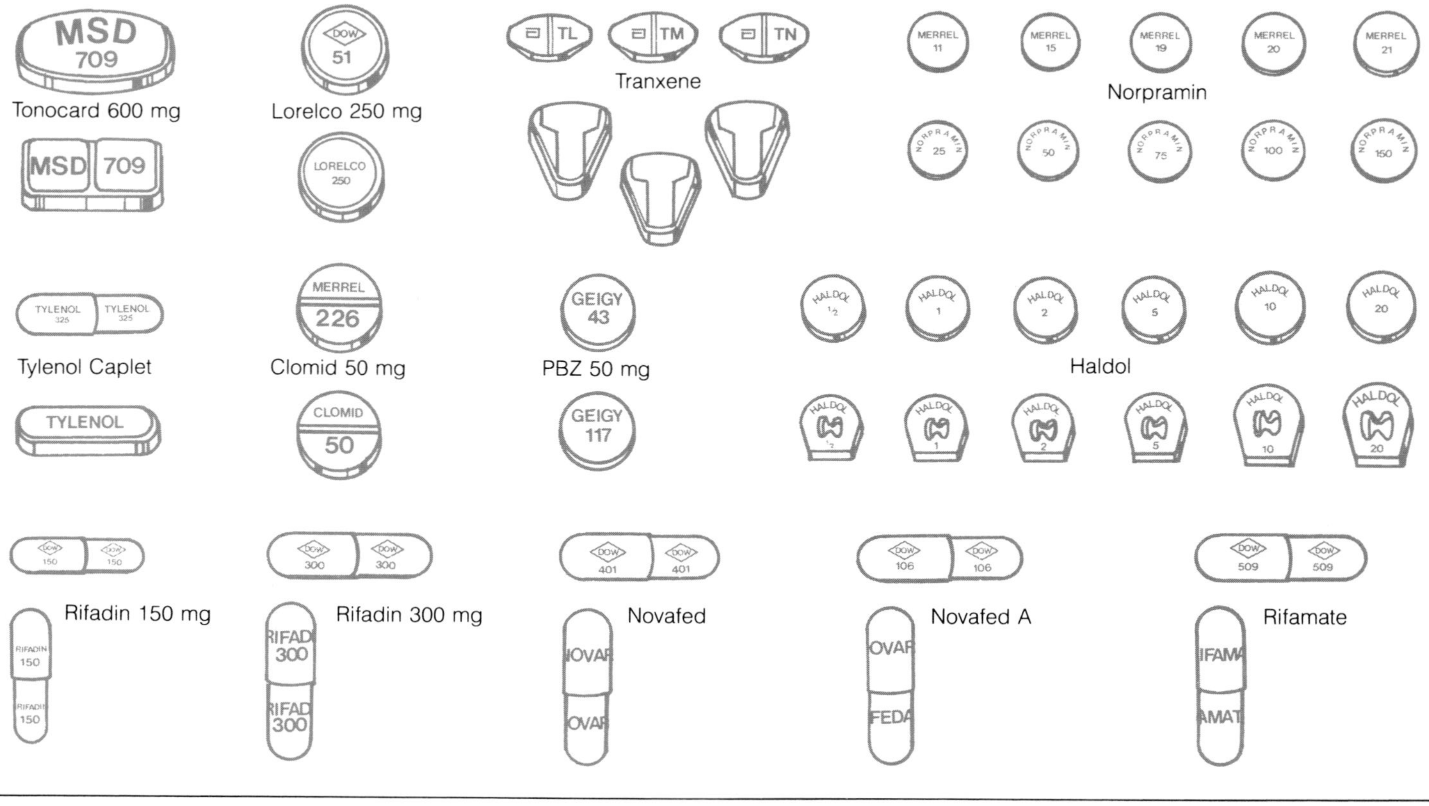

Tonocard 600 mg

Lorelco 250 mg

Tranxene

Norpramin

Tylenol Caplet

Clomid 50 mg

PBZ 50 mg

Haldol

Rifadin 150 mg

Rifadin 300 mg

Novafed

Novafed A

Rifamate

Medication administration

Caring for a patient who needs long-term I.V. medication administration? Depending on his condition and on the drug he needs, he now has more options than ever before. New administration devices and techniques available today enhance therapy while helping to preserve the patient's independence.

Take subcutaneous venous access devices, for example. Protected by a skin barrier, these implanted devices provide I.V. access without repeated venipunctures—a blessing for a patient who needs long-term intermittent therapy. Similarly, an implantable pump provides continuous I.V. medication infusions without disturbing the patient's life-style or body image.

If your patient needs relief from acute or intractable chronic pain, the doctor may order patient-controlled analgesia with a special pump the patient controls himself (with some limitations). With pain relief at his fingertips, the patient will probably achieve better pain control with less narcotic than if he depended on you for periodic injections.

In the following pages, we'll also acquaint you with metered-dose inhalers and a new reusable syringe that simplifies administration of some injectable drugs.

Learning about subcutaneous venous access devices

Designed primarily for patients needing long-term or intermittent treatment with an I.V. medication, a subcutaneous venous access device provides I.V. access without repeated venipunctures. Because all its components lie under the skin (in contrast to a Hickman or Broviac catheter, which has an external portion), it doesn't need a dressing and won't disturb the patient's body image or interfere with his activities. When not in use, it needs heparinization only about once a month, not daily. However, also unlike a Hickman catheter, it requires skin puncture for access.

The Cormed Mediport device shown below includes a self-sealing silicone rubber injection port that maintains its integrity for up to 2,000 punctures. Shaped like a volcano, the stainless-steel reservoir body has a Dacron mesh base for patient comfort. *Note:* Cormed also makes a similar two-port device.

To implant the device, the doctor hollows a subcutaneous pocket—typically, in the upper chest—for the injection port and reservoir. He then creates a subcutaneous tunnel and threads the catheter through it into a central vein. Finally, he sutures the port to underlying fascia, flushes the device with heparin, and closes the incision. Fluoroscopy or an X-ray confirms proper placement. The procedure, usually performed with a local anesthetic, takes an hour or less. *Note:* As needed, the device can be implanted anywhere in the body and can provide access to any vessel or cavity, including the epidural space, the peritoneal cavity, and the hepatic artery. For maximum stability, the port should overlie a bony structure—for example, the clavicle.

You can palpate the device easily once it's in place. Depending on the amount of tissue covering it, you may see a slight protrusion at the site.

To preserve the injection port's integrity, use *only* noncoring Huber needles to puncture it. Standard needles hollow out silicone, destroying the port's ability to reseal. For more on using a Mediport device, read the photostory on page 66.

Mediport Implantable Vascular Access Port

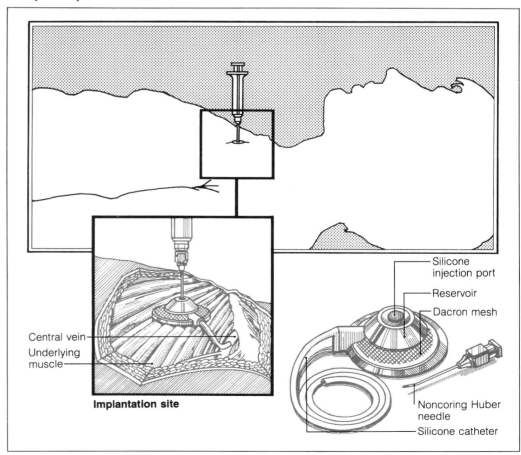

Central vein
Underlying muscle
Implantation site

Silicone injection port
Reservoir
Dacron mesh
Noncoring Huber needle
Silicone catheter

Medication administration

Using Mediport to give a bolus injection

The following photostory illustrates the basic procedure for using an implanted venous access system to give a bolus injection. Read the photostory on page 67 for some special considerations that apply to giving a continuous infusion and withdrawing a blood specimen. Note: Some details (such as the amount of saline flush solution to use) differ from hospital to hospital.

For patients who object to the pain of skin puncture, the doctor may order a local anesthetic (such as lidocaine) for subcutaneous injection before Huber needle insertion.

Before using the device to administer medication or withdraw blood, confirm proper catheter placement with an X-ray. Some patients consciously or unconsciously manipulate implanted equipment—a phenomenon (called Twiddler's syndrome) *that was first observed among patients with pacemakers. An X-ray verifies that the catheter remains in position.*

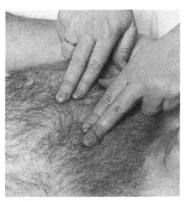

1 Gather povidone-iodine swabs, a needle and syringe containing 3 to 5 ml heparin solution (100 units/ml), a 10-ml syringe (with needle) containing sterile saline solution, a Huber needle, 6″ (5 cm) I.V. extension tubing, and medication. (Hospital policy may also require sterile gloves.)
Wash your hands and position the patient comfortably. Palpate to locate the reservoir and injection port.

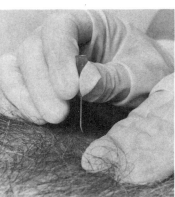

2 Prepare the site, according to hospital policy. Stabilize the Mediport reservoir between your thumb and forefinger. Hold the Huber needle like a dart, and position it at a 90-degree angle over the septum, as shown here. Push it straight through the skin and septum until you feel it hit the needle stop at the back of the septum. (Don't insert the needle at an angle, or you may damage the septum.)

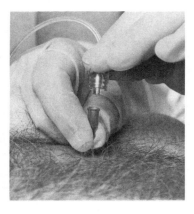

3 Attach the extension tubing to the needle hub. *Note:* As an alternative, you can attach a stopcock to the needle hub. However, extension tubing maintains a closed system for drug administration and other uses while minimizing needle manipulation.

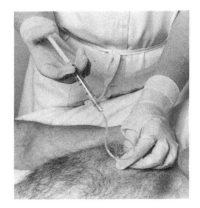

4 Steadily inject 5 ml saline flush solution. If you can't inject the solution, the Huber needle tip may be malpositioned. Make sure you've advanced it to the needle stop and again try to inject the solution. If you still fail, remove the Huber needle and start over.

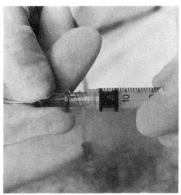

5 After injecting the saline flush solution, remove the needle and syringe. Then inject the ordered medication into the extension tubing port. Flush the tubing with 5 ml saline solution. *Important:* To prevent problems from drug incompatibilities, flush the device with saline solution before and after each drug injection and before each heparinization.

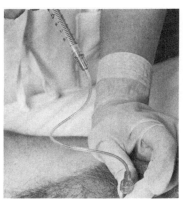

6 Flush the tubing with 3 to 5 ml heparin solution, according to policy. *Note:* While in regular use, the Mediport doesn't need any additional heparin flushing. However, when not in use, it should be flushed once a month to maintain patency.

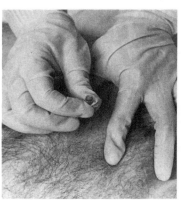

7 To remove the Huber needle, stabilize the reservoir between your thumb and forefinger. Then withdraw the needle, taking care not to twist or angle it. After needle withdrawal, you may see a slight amount of serosanguineous discharge at the puncture site.

Giving a continuous infusion: Special considerations

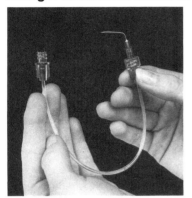

1 To give a continuous infusion of medication, fluids, blood, or blood products, use extension tubing with a Luer-Lok and clamp and a right-angled Huber needle (see photo). Cleanse the insertion site and prime the I.V. tubing.

Using sterile technique, insert the needle. Stabilize it at its hub to prevent rotation.

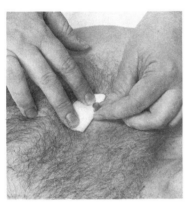

2 After insertion, the needle's upper portion should lie just above the skin surface. If it lies more than 0.5 cm above the surface, support it with a folded 2″ × 2″ gauze pad, as shown here.

Use sterile adhesive strips to secure first the needle hub, then the extension tubing. Apply povidone-iodine ointment to the insertion site. Then apply a sterile transparent dressing, such as the Cormed Port Gard.

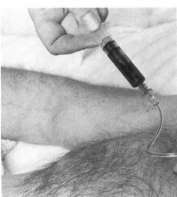

3 To withdraw a blood specimen after starting the infusion, close the extension tubing clamp, disconnect and cap the I.V. tubing, and attach a 5-ml syringe. Withdraw and discard 3 to 5 ml blood; then withdraw a specimen into a new syringe or (if you're using a Vacutainer adapter) into Vacutainer tubes. (For problem-solving strategies, see the troubleshooting tips at right.)

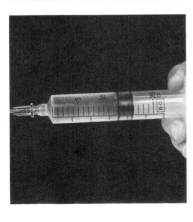

4 Inject 10 to 20 ml normal saline flush solution to clear the system, then restart the infusion. (Or, if the infusion's complete, heparinize the device and remove the Huber needle.)

For long-term therapy, a Huber needle can remain in place for 7 to 10 days at a time. Regularly inspect the site for signs of infiltration, infection, and irritation. Change dressings according to hospital policy.

Clots and other occlusions: Troubleshooting tips

If you have trouble withdrawing blood from a Mediport device—even though you can easily inject flush solution and an X-ray confirms proper catheter placement—the catheter tip may be resting against the vessel wall. Try changing the patient's position. Or ask him to bear down (Valsalva's maneuver) while you try to jog the catheter tip by alternating saline flushes with attempts to aspirate.

Fibrin sheath formation
Over time, some catheters develop a fibrin sheath. Aspiration sucks the sheath into the tip, temporarily occluding it. If fluoroscopy confirms sheath formation, continue to use the device to infuse fluids, but obtain blood specimens from another site. The doctor probably won't replace the device because sheath formation tends to recur in susceptible patients.

Clotting problems
If permitted by hospital policy, you can solve some clotting problems easily by heparinizing the catheter and leaving it alone for about 45 minutes. Or, if the needle's occluded with minute fibrin particles, a needle change may solve the problem. If these simple measures don't work, however, the doctor may attempt to alternately aspirate and irrigate the catheter. *Important:* Always obtain a large-volume syringe for this procedure. A small syringe may exert too much pressure and rupture the catheter.

If aspiration/irrigation fails, administer a fibrinolytic agent (streptokinase or urokinase), as ordered, using a tuberculin syringe. Attempt to aspirate the clot after 10 minutes. Repeat the procedure at 5-minute intervals, as necessary.

Medication administration

Learning about the Infusaid implantable pump

Harry Black, a 66-year-old retired teacher, learned a year ago that he has colon cancer. Recently his doctor told him that the cancer has spread to his liver. To treat the metastasis, his doctor orders treatment with floxuridine (FUDR), an antineoplastic drug infused directly into the hepatic artery. To allow Mr. Black to remain active during therapy, the doctor recommends administering the drug via an implantable pump. After Mr. Black learns more about it, he agrees.

The Infusaid implantable pump featured here is a palm-sized device powered by a bellows system (see illustration at right). Models have one or two side ports, which permit bolus injections, injection of radiopaque dye, and supplemental infusions. A dual-catheter model permits the doctor to treat two different sites or to provide a combination of local and systemic therapy.

During the insertion procedure, the doctor places the pump's catheter in the targeted organ or vessel—in Mr. Black's case, the hepatic artery. He sutures the pump into a subcutaneous pocket created in chest or abdominal tissue (depending on the catheter site). The pump then delivers precise drug doses from its drug reservoir directly to the target area, permitting more effective drug delivery with fewer systemic side effects. For regional chemotherapy, areas the pump treats include the liver, head, neck, and central nervous system (CNS).

The pump has no external catheters or exit sites—a feature that minimizes infection risks. Consequently, it requires no dressing or special care. Because the reservoir can be refilled by injection in the doctor's office, the patient can remain ambulatory during therapy.

Besides floxuridine, the Infusaid pump can deliver fluorouracil (5-FU), methotrexate, morphine, amikacin, heparin, glycerol, saline solution, and bacteriostatic water. Other drugs under study for pump administration include antibiotics for osteomyelitis treatment, drugs to treat CNS disorders, and additional antineoplastic drugs.

Infusaid implantable pump

The pump's design provides a virtually unlimited power source. When the inner chamber—the drug reservoir—fills with fluid, the bellows expand. The bellows, in turn, compress the outer chamber, which contains a two-phase charging fluid. During drug administration, the patient's body temperature warms the charging fluid, causing it to expand and compress the bellows. The bellows then force the drug through a bacterial membrane filter and preset flow restrictor. Preset flow rates range from 1 to 6 ml/day, and reservoir capacity ranges from 22 to 47 ml (depending on the pump model).

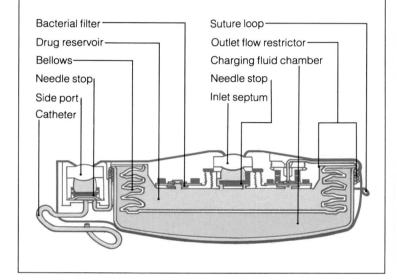

Bacterial filter
Drug reservoir
Bellows
Needle stop
Side port
Catheter

Suture loop
Outlet flow restrictor
Charging fluid chamber
Needle stop
Inlet septum

SPECIAL CONSIDERATIONS

Points to remember about Infusaid

To ensure safe, effective drug therapy, keep these special considerations in mind.

How to maintain accurate flow rates

Refill the Infusaid pump with only the drugs (or fluids) it's designed to deliver. Flow rate has been factory-set. Refer to the Infusaid Pump Performance Data Sheet packaged with the pump for details on dosage and infusion volume.

To ensure dosage accuracy throughout therapy, remember that these factors affect flow rate:
• *atmospheric pressure*. At high altitudes (and during airplane travel), reduced atmospheric pressure increases flow rate.
• *body temperature*. Above 98.6° F. (37° C.), drug flow increases 10% to 13% for each 1-degree rise. A temperature drop reduces flow rate proportionately.
• *blood pressure*. Flow rate diminishes 3% for each 10 mm Hg that average arterial blood pressure rises above 90 mm Hg. Flow rate rises in the same proportions when average arterial blood pressure drops below 90 mm Hg.

• *drug concentration and viscosity*. Some drugs, such as heparin, have concentration-dependent viscosities that affect flow rate. Consult the Performance Data Sheet for guidance.

What to tell the patient

Teach your patient how his pump functions and how to avoid problems. For example, tell him to:
• avoid contact sports
• consult his doctor before traveling by plane or visiting high altitudes
• avoid deep-sea diving and scuba diving
• avoid long, hot baths and saunas
• report fever to his doctor immediately
• report any unusual symptoms related to drug therapy
• keep all appointments for drug refills
• carry an Infusaid patient identification card.

How to refill an Infusaid pump

Besides teaching your patient about his pump, your biggest responsibility may be refilling the pump's drug reservoir. After reviewing the pump's manual, use this photostory as a guide. Note: Also check policy to make sure that refilling an implantable pump is a nursing responsibility in your hospital. Some hospitals require special certification.

Obtain an Infusaid Refill Kit, which includes a 50-ml syringe barrel (you won't need a plunger), fillset tubing with stopcock (1-ml capacity), special Infusaid needles, iodine and alcohol swabs, gauze pads, a drape, a pump template, and an adhesive bandage strip. In addition, gather sterile gloves, a 5-ml syringe filled with sterile water, a 50-ml syringe (for drug administration), and the ordered drug. Make sure the drug is warm (62° to 95° F. [15° to 35° C.]).

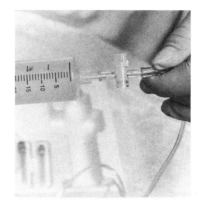

4 Attach the 50-ml syringe barrel (shown here) and the Infusaid needle to the fillset. Tighten all connections.

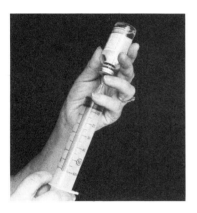

1 Fill the 50-ml syringe with the warmed drug. *Note:* Only Infusaid pump models 100 and 400 have a 50-ml drug capacity. If you're using another model, consult the manual for instructions.

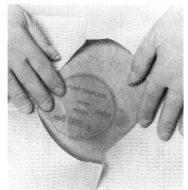

5 To help you locate the septum, place the template cover over the pump, as shown here. (However, if you can palpate the septum easily, you may prefer to skip this step.)

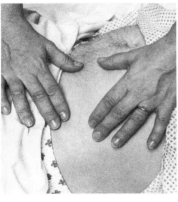

2 Wash your hands; then gently palpate the pump to find its perimeter. Next, find the inlet septum, located near the pump's center and indented about ¼". *Important:* Don't rely on puncture marks from previous refills; the skin may have shifted slightly over the pump.

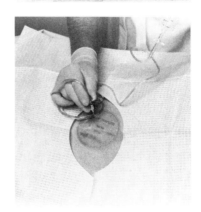

6 Insert the Infusaid needle into the septum at a perpendicular angle. (Use only Infusaid needles to puncture the septum.)

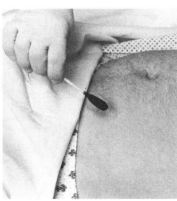

3 Open the sterile Refill Kit, don sterile gloves, prepare the pump site (as shown), and drape the area.

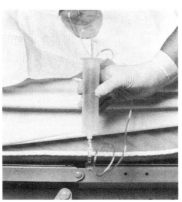

7 Open the fillset stopcock. Then position the syringe barrel below the pump and allow the pump to empty. *Caution:* Never aspirate fluid from the pump; aspiration may draw blood into the catheter and cause an occlusion.

Medication administration

How to refill an Infusaid pump continued

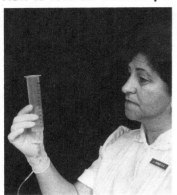

8 Note the volume of returned fluid. (Add 1 ml to the volume collected in the syringe barrel to account for fluid in the fillset tubing.)
If no fluid returns, remove the syringe barrel and replace it with a 5-ml syringe filled with sterile water. Inject the water and wait for fluid to return. If necessary, repeat the procedure once. If no fluid returns, stop the procedure and report the problem. Pump failure may be responsible.

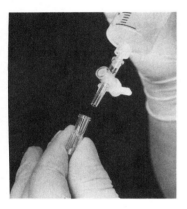

9 Close the stopcock; then remove and discard the syringe barrel and stopcock. Leave the needle and fillset in place.

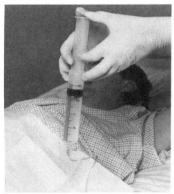

10 Attach the drug-filled syringe to the fillset. Then inject 5 ml of drug into the pump, using both hands, as shown.

11 Reconfirm proper needle placement by releasing pressure on the plunger and looking for drug return in the syringe. Then inject the remaining drug in 5-ml increments, rechecking needle placement between increments. After you've injected the ordered dose, quickly pull out the needle, remove the template, cleanse iodine from the patient's skin, and apply an adhesive bandage strip.

Giving a bolus dose through the Infusaid side port

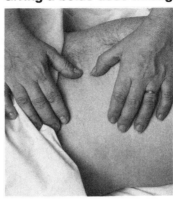

1 Gather this equipment: an Infusaid Fillset Kit, two 5-ml syringes filled with sterile water, a syringe filled with the drug dose, and sterile gloves. *Note:* Use only 3- to 5-ml syringes for side port injection. Wash your hands. Palpate to locate the pump's perimeter, inlet septum, and side port.

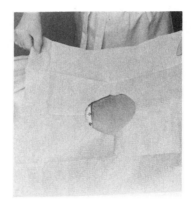

2 Don gloves; then prepare and drape the site.

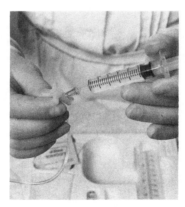

3 Attach the syringe filled with sterile water to the Infusaid needle and fillset, as shown. Tighten all connections and close the stopcock.

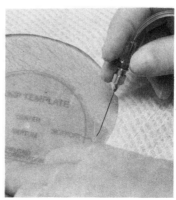

4 Insert the Infusaid needle into the side port septum at a perpendicular angle.

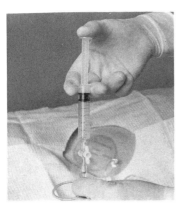

5 Open the stopcock and inject the water to flush the catheter. Release pressure on the syringe plunger. Then close the stopcock and remove and discard the syringe.

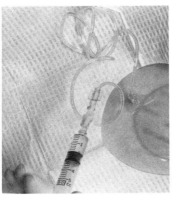

6 Next, attach the drug-filled syringe to the fillset and open the stopcock. Slowly inject the drug. *Caution:* Limit the injection rate to 10 ml over 10 minutes to avoid increasing the pressure.

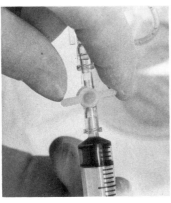

7 After injecting the drug, close the stopcock (as shown) and remove the syringe. Attach the second syringe of sterile water to the fillset, open the stopcock, and flush the catheter.

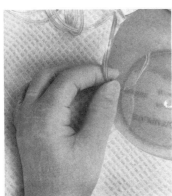

8 Close the stopcock and withdraw the needle from the side port, as shown. Remove the template, cleanse iodine from the patient's skin, if necessary, and apply the adhesive bandage strip.

Learning about patient-controlled analgesia

Patient-controlled analgesia (PCA) puts pain relief at the patient's fingertips. At the patient's initiation, a preprogrammed PCA pump releases narcotic doses within preset limits. It can also periodically release small narcotic doses into the patient's bloodstream at a preset basal rate.

Besides sparing the patient repeated I.M. injections, PCA pumps provide a constant plateau of analgesia, usually without causing undue drowsiness or respiratory depression. Studies show that compared to patients receiving I.M. narcotic injections, those using a pump need less narcotic to control pain, develop fewer postoperative complications, and ambulate sooner.

Indications and contraindications

The doctor may order a pump for any patient with an I.V. line who suffers from acute postoperative pain or severe intractable pain; for example, from traumatic injury or from a chronic condition such as cancer. For best results, the patient should also be alert and mentally competent. Poor candidates for pump therapy include known or suspected drug abusers, patients with respiratory disease, severely debilitated patients, and the elderly. *Caution:* Correct acute hypovolemia before initiating pump therapy.

The Harvard PCA

A computerized pump, the Bard Harvard PCA pictured on page 72 runs on wall power but includes a battery backup for operation during transport or power failure. It operates in three modes: PCA (for patient-controlled bolus injections only), PCA/basal (for patient-controlled boluses plus a continuous basal infusion given automatically), and continuous infusion (for continuous infusion of I.V. fluids and drugs). Safety features, including a side-mounted lock and programmable security code, prevent unauthorized access. The Harvard PCA also has a dose-delay period, during which the pump won't give the patient a requested bolus injection. Other features include:
• a 1-hour dosage limit period, which prevents the pump from delivering more than a programmed maximum dose within an hour.
• an automatic memory that records how many times the patient requests medication during the delay period and how many doses the pump delivers.
• an ATTENTION indicator light that signals improper operating conditions and a display panel that explains the problem.

Examine the photos on the next few pages to learn how to set up the Harvard PCA.

Medication administration

Harvard PCA pump

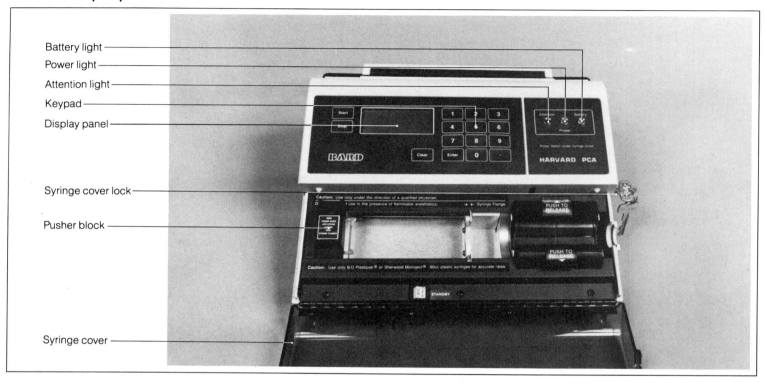

Battery light
Power light
Attention light
Keypad
Display panel
Syringe cover lock
Pusher block
Syringe cover

Setting up the Harvard PCA

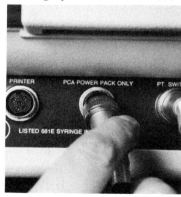

1 This photostory demonstrates the set-up for the PCA or PCA/basal mode. See the following photostory for details on the continuous infusion mode.
Install the pump's fuse, the patient switch plug, and the power pack connector, as directed by the manufacturer. *Note:* Normally, you'd place the pump on an I.V. pole platform. For demonstration purposes, however, we've placed it on a bedside table.

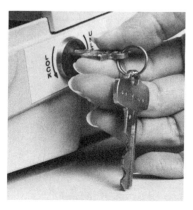

2 To lock the pump to the I.V. pole platform, unlock and open the syringe cover (see photo). Use a screwdriver to tighten the two captive fasteners—one located to the left of the drive mechanism, the other above the closed syringe holder on the right.

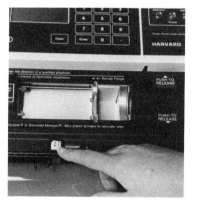

3 Turn on the pump. The display panel will briefly flash this message: RAM-OK CTC-OK INT-OK RTC-OK ROM-OK. When the message disappears, you should hear a beep and see the message SELF TEST COMPLETE (the green POWER light should also come on). If you see any other message on the display panel, consult the operator's manual for troubleshooting instructions.

4 Fill a syringe with the ordered drug. *Important:* Use only 60-ml B-D Plastipak or 60-ml Sherwood Monoject plastic Luer-Lok syringes with the Harvard PCA.

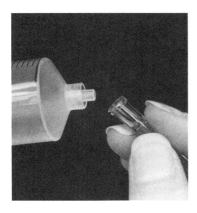

5 Attach a Harvard Microbore 60" or 96" Tamperproof Extension Set to the syringe, as shown, and flush air from the system.

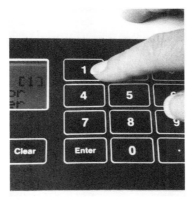

9 Now, flush the tubing by pressing and holding the 1 key, as shown here, until fluid emerges from the tubing.

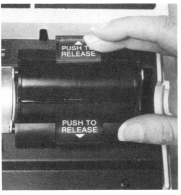

6 To install the syringe in the pump, squeeze the pusher block release and slide the block to the extreme left. Prepare the syringe cradle to receive the syringe by spreading the PUSH TO RELEASE tabs, as shown here.

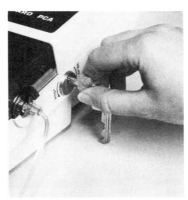

10 Close the syringe cover and turn the syringe cover key counterclockwise to lock the cover.

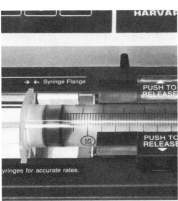

7 Lay the syringe barrel in the cradle, aligning the barrel flange with the syringe flange slots. Press down on the syringe barrel, so that the cradle segments move to the locked position.

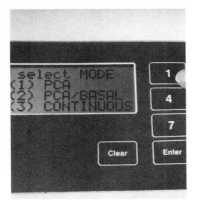

11 Select the infusion mode. Press the 1 key to select the PCA mode, the 2 key to select the PCA/basal mode, or the 3 key to select the continuous infusion mode. Next, prepare the primary infusion line. If the patient already has an I.V. line in place, disconnect the line from him, install the Bard Anti-Reflux Microbore Y-Set, flush the tubing, and reconnect the line. Then connect the syringe extension set's distal end to the Y-Set.

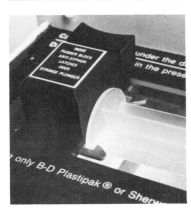

8 Squeeze the pusher block release and advance the block to the right, until its anti-siphon latches enclose the syringe plunger flange, as shown here. The pusher block should press firmly against the syringe plunger.

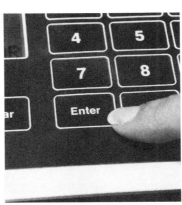

12 After you press the 1 key (PCA mode) or the 2 key (PCA/basal mode), you'll see a date and time on the display panel. If they're correct, press ENTER.

Medication administration

Setting up the Harvard PCA continued

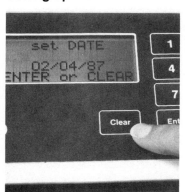

13 If they're not correct, press CLEAR. Select values as directed on the display screen. *Note:* Don't forget to enter leading zeros, if necessary.

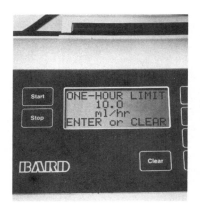

17 The display now shows the default 1-hour dosage limit: 10 ml/hour. If this is acceptable, press ENTER. However, if the doctor has ordered a different limit, reprogram the dosage limit by pressing the appropriate numbers. (Programmable range: 0.1 to 30 ml/hour.)

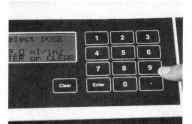

14 Program the drug dose per injection (as ordered) by pressing the appropriate keypad numbers, then pressing ENTER. (If you make a mistake during any portion of the programming process, press CLEAR and start again.) The maximum dose you can program is 9.9 ml.

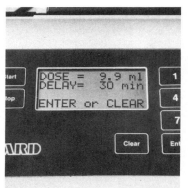

18 The display window now shows each value you've entered. Press ENTER to confirm that the value is correct. If a value isn't correct, press CLEAR and enter the correct value.

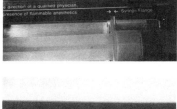

15 Next, select the delay time between injections (the interval during which the pump won't respond to patient requests). You can program any delay from 3 to 60 minutes, as ordered. Press the appropriate numbers, then press ENTER.

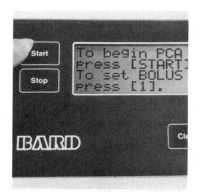

19 Press START to begin PCA or PCA/basal operation. Or press the 1 key to provide a bolus injection.

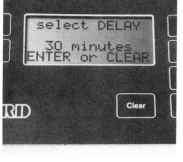

16 If the doctor ordered PCA with a basal flow rate and you pressed the 2 key in Step 11, you should now enter the basal flow rate. The pump can deliver a maximum basal dosage of 10 ml/hour.

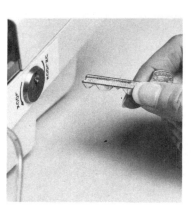

20 Remove the key from the syringe cover lock to guard against tampering. *Note:* Consult the operator's manual for information on giving an optional loading dose.

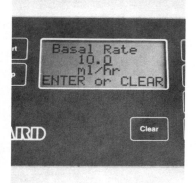

Giving a continuous infusion with the Harvard PCA

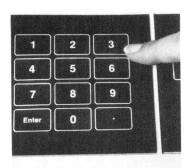

1 Set up the pump, as shown in Steps 1 through 11 in the previous photostory. Choose the continuous infusion mode by pressing the 3 key.

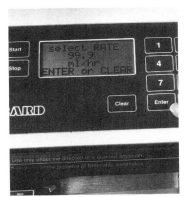

2 To program the ordered flow rate, press the appropriate keypad numbers, followed by ENTER. (The pump can deliver up to 99.9 ml/hour.) Then program infusion volume by pressing the appropriate keypad numbers (to a maximum of 99.9 ml), followed by ENTER. The display window shows the two values you've entered. If they're correct, press ENTER. To make a correction, press CLEAR and reenter the values.

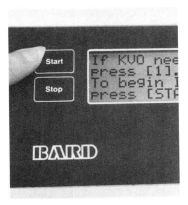

3 Set up an I.V. line in the normal manner and attach it to the patient. Connect the pump syringe's extension tubing to the Bard Anti-Reflux Microbore Y-Set. Then begin the infusion by pressing START. (The pump can also deliver an infusion at a keep-vein-open flow rate. Consult the operator's manual for instructions.)

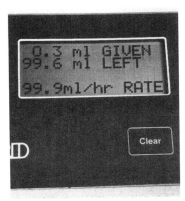

4 Throughout the infusion, the display window shows the volume delivered, the volume remaining, and the flow rate. The pump delivers fluid until the syringe empties or you press STOP. After stopping the infusion, press START to restart the infusion, saving all data; or CLEAR to cancel previously programmed data.

Using a Tubex Fast-Trak Syringe

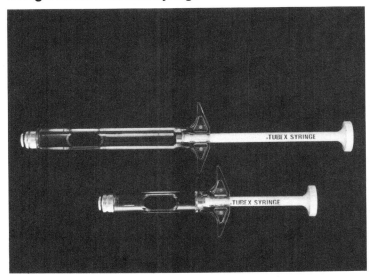

Use a Tubex Fast-Trak Syringe to administer medications or heparinized flush solution from a disposable cartridge-needle unit (which consists of a prefilled medication vial, needle, and needle guard). As shown in the photo above, the reusable plastic and stainless-steel syringe comes in two sizes: 1 ml and 2 ml. To use the equipment, follow these steps:

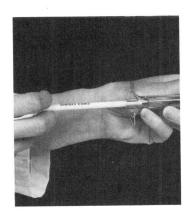

1 First, withdraw the syringe plunger as far as possible.

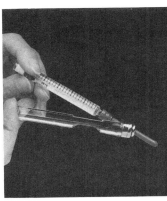

2 Insert the ordered Tubex Sterile Cartridge-Needle Unit, needle-end first.

Medication administration

Using a Tubex Fast-Trak Syringe continued

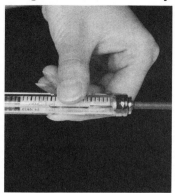

3 To engage the needle hub and cartridge, rotate the cartridge clockwise. You'll hear a clicking noise when the cartridge engages fully.

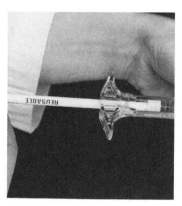

4 Next, gently rotate the plunger clockwise until the cartridge turns with the plunger.

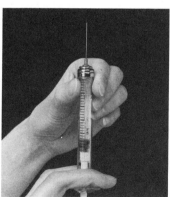

5 Pull off the needle guard and expel air, as shown here. Then inject the medication into the patient or his I.V. injection port.
    After giving the injection, replace the needle guard, unscrew and withdraw the plunger, and rotate the cartridge counterclockwise to disengage the front end.

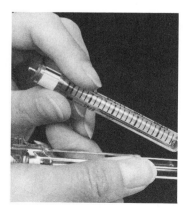

6 Remove the empty cartridge, and dispose of the cartridge and needle according to hospital policy.

Using a metered-dose inhaler

For a patient with chronic respiratory disease, a metered-dose inhaler (MDI) provides a more effective alternative to hand-held nebulizers. The self-contained MDI unit consists of an inhaler attached to a unit-dose pressurized canister or capsule containing bronchodilators or steroids (see box on page 77). The doctor may prescribe an MDI to treat chronic respiratory disease or acute conditions such as asthma attacks.
    To use an MDI effectively, the patient must synchronize medication delivery with inhalations. If she can't—for example, because she has arthritis—she may need an extender (or spacer) to delay medication delivery (see the procedure shown at right).
    After you teach your patient to use an MDI (see following illustrations), she can use it independently at home.

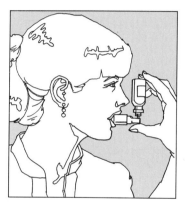

1 First, instruct your patient to shake the MDI well, so that the medication and aerosol propellant mix. Then have her exhale fully and place the MDI mouthpiece between her lips. Tell her to make sure neither her tongue nor her teeth block the opening. *Note:* Some doctors recommend the open-mouth technique: the patient opens her mouth wide and positions the mouthpiece 2″ to 4″ from her lips.

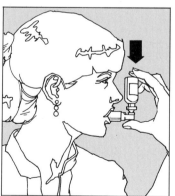

2 Now, instruct the patient to press down on the canister while beginning a slow, deep inhalation. Inhaling slowly and deeply ensures maximum medication delivery. (Your patient may need practice to master this step.) *Note:* If your patient's using the open-mouth technique, have her release medication at the beginning of an inhalation that lasts about 5 seconds.

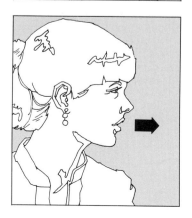

3 After she has inhaled fully, tell her to hold her breath for 10 seconds, then to slowly exhale through her nose or pursed lips.
    If the doctor has ordered two doses, have the patient wait 2 minutes and repeat the procedure.

Using an InspirEase extender

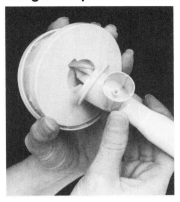

1 Using valves or a reservoir bag, an extender delays medication delivery for patients who can't master MDI technique. The extenders currently available fit most MDIs. These photos show how to use the InspirEase extender, which has a reservoir bag.

The patient connects the mouthpiece to the reservoir bag by lining up the inhaler's locking tabs with the bag's opening, as shown.

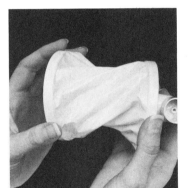

2 Next, she gently untwists the reservoir bag to open it fully. After shaking the MDI, she places it snugly in the mouthpiece holder.

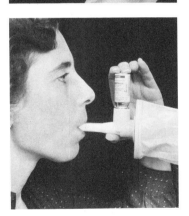

3 She places the extender mouthpiece in her mouth and closes her lips tightly around it. Then, to release medication into the bag, she presses down on the MDI canister once or twice, as ordered.

Next, she inhales slowly through the mouthpiece. *Note:* Tell her that if she hears a whistling sound, she's inhaling too quickly.

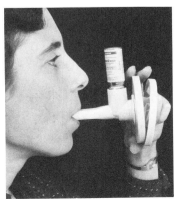

4 She continues inhaling until the bag collapses. Then she holds her breath for 5 seconds and breathes out slowly into the bag.

As ordered, she repeats the entire procedure.

Brethancer: Designed for convenience

One of the newest extenders on the market, Brethancer consists of three interlocking plastic components that telescope together for convenient carrying between uses. Easily opened in one motion, the device traps medication in its middle portion for the patient to inhale.

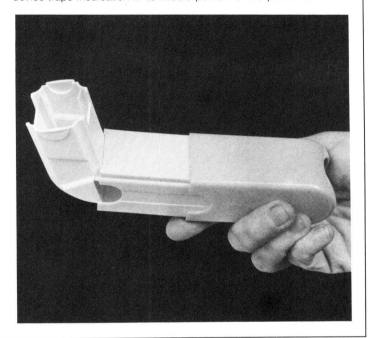

UPDATE

Drugs delivered by MDI: Some examples

Bronchodilators
- albuterol (Proventil, Ventolin)
- bitolterol (Tornalate)
- epinephrine (Medihaler-Epi, Primatene Mist)
- isoetharine (Bronkometer)
- isoproterenol (Isuprel, Medihaler-Iso)
- metaproterenol (Alupent, Metaprel)
- terbutaline (Brethaire)

Corticosteroids for oral inhalation
- beclomethasone (Beclovent, Vanceril)
- flunisolide (AeroBid)
- triamcinolone (Azmacort)

I.V. therapy

The equipment we feature in the following pages can help you with one of your most important nursing responsibilities—managing I.V. therapy. The sophisticated Omni-Flow 4000 pump, for example, can deliver up to four drugs continuously or intermittently, depending on your patient's needs. We also feature:

- the Controlled Release Infusion System for secondary drug administration
- the multiple-lumen central venous catheter, which can deliver up to four infusions through separate lumens inside the catheter
- the Vena-Vue Vein Evaluator for locating hard-to-find veins.

Using the Omni-Flow 4000 infusion pump

Your patient's receiving several I.V. drugs. Throughout your shift, you administer antibiotics every 4 hours, monitor a lipid infusion, inject a furosemide bolus, and frequently check I.V. lines for patency. Imagine how much time you'd save if a pump could take over some of these functions.

The Omni-Flow 4000 (shown below), a computerized infusion pump attached to a single administration set, performs all these functions and more. You'll appreciate its versatility and built-in safety features.

Pump design and functions

Designed to deliver up to four drugs continuously or intermittently, the piston-driven Omni-Flow 4000 runs on wall power or battery power for up to 5 hours. Its cassette has Luer-Lok connectors that attach to special primary and secondary sets large enough to infuse blood, packed cells, and lipid emulsions. You can also connect 10-ml (or larger) syringes to the cassette. A small collection bag on the primary set eliminates air bubbles from the cassette.

An I.V. pole available from the manufacturer provides a mounting base for the pump and a four-bottle hanger. The pole's offset design stabilizes the 13-lb pump. (If you use a standard I.V. pole, attach the pump and I.V. containers with special care.)

The pump's front panel contains a back-lit display screen that shows programming messages, a line status panel that reports dosage and remaining volume for each line, and an easy-to-use keyboard for programming delivery rates and times. You can also program the pump to perform these functions:

- infuse up to four continuous I.V.s at the ordered rate
- maintain a keep-vein-open I.V. rate of between 1.4 and 99.9 ml/hour
- stop a continuous infusion while other lines deliver intermittent doses (when the primary line is in the maintenance mode)
- dilute and infuse single drug doses
- infuse a drug intermittently for 24 hours
- change I.V. line occlusion pressures
- put all lines on hold while you obtain pressure readings
- sound an alarm if problems develop
- stop or reset any or all lines
- flush or cancel flushes between intermittent infusions.

Safety features

Whenever it's on, the pump performs a self-test of electrical and mechanical components. It maintains a duplicate memory of programmed information and sounds an alarm if a discrepancy occurs. You can't accidentally change programmed information, because each change requires two entries. And, as long as the cassette's locked, no I.V. free flow or drug overdose can occur.

When problems or changes occur anywhere in the system, the pump's alarm sounds. The display screen indicates the problem and corrective action. When infusing intermittent drugs, you can set the call-back alarm to alert you when drug administration starts and finishes. This feature helps you monitor the patient's response to treatment.

Now read the following photostory to learn how to perform the pump's basic operations. Before using the pump, refer to the manufacturer's operations manual; use the compact operations guide for quick bedside reference. The manual also provides instructions for special pump functions.

Omni-Flow 4000

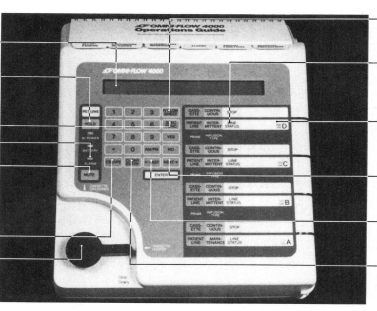

Display screen.

Hold key. Puts operating lines on hold for up to 2 minutes.

Special functions key. Permits you to program a special pump function.

Alarm light.

Mute key.

Escape key. When pressed, calls up the pump status screen in the display window. Allows you to start over if you make a mistake programming.

Cassette locking lever.

I.V. flow sheet key. Calls up a running total of volume infused by each line and a total of all four lines.

Line function panel. Consists of six keys; provides current programming information for each line. (Information appears on the display screen.)

Line indicator light. Glows continuously when you program a line to start; blinks when the line is operating.

Next key. Moves the programming cursor to the next information entry point on the screen.

Last key. Moves the cursor to the last information entry point on the screen.

Clear entry key. Changes the information at the entry point where the cursor appears back to its original value.

Setting up the Omni-Flow 4000 primary line

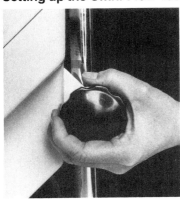

1 First, clamp the pump securely to an I.V. pole. Make sure the display screen is visible and the keyboard accessible. Plug the cord into a wall outlet.

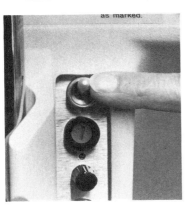

2 Next, locate the pump's power compartment in the back. Pull the safety switch out and up to turn the power on. Note the green light on the display panel (AC PWR). All other lights should be off.

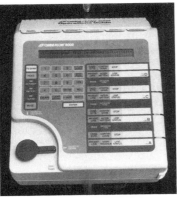

3 Observe the display screen. It reads *SELF TEST IN PROGRESS* while the pump performs a 6-second test for malfunctions.

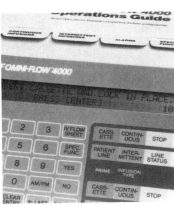

4 If the pump checks out properly, you'll see the first programming message on the display screen: *INSERT CASSETTE AND LOCK IN PLACE. PRESS [ENTER].* This message remains on the screen until you insert the cassette (see Step 9).

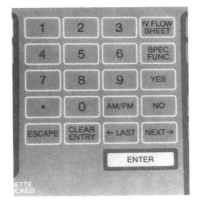

5 The time appears in the display screen's lower right corner. Use the keyboard shown here to set the correct time.

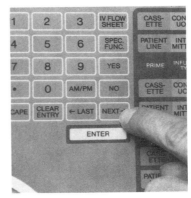

6 To make an AM or PM change, press the NEXT key once to move the cursor. Press the AM/PM key, then the ENTER key.

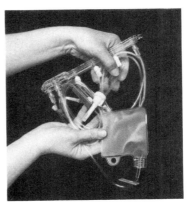

7 Remove the Omni-Flow 4000 Primary Pump Set from the package. You'll see that the primary infusion tubing (Line A), air collection bag, and patient line are attached to the cassette. Close the upper clamp on Line A and tighten the cassette's Luer-Lok connectors.

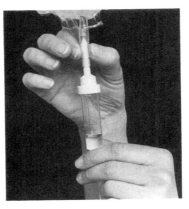

8 Attach the tubing to the I.V. container and hang the container on the pole. Squeeze the drip chamber. *Important:* Make sure the I.V. solution is compatible with the medications in the secondary I.V. lines. Carefully check all medication labels against the doctor's order and the patient's I.V. before beginning infusions.

I.V. therapy

Setting up the Omni-Flow 4000 primary line continued

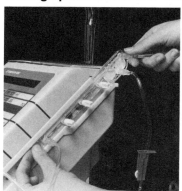

9 Now, open the cassette locking lever. Grasp the cassette, keeping the patient line and the collection bag at the top. Insert the cassette into the holster on the pump's right side. Make sure connectors point to your right, as shown in the photo. *Note:* The pump's power must be on to engage the cassette.

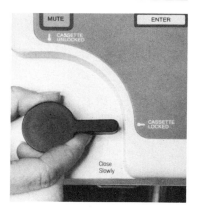

10 Lock the cassette by turning the cassette locking lever clockwise, as shown. Then open the I.V. clamps and check to make sure that no fluid flows into the drip chamber. *Caution:* Take care to lock the cassette before opening the clamps, or fluid will flow freely.

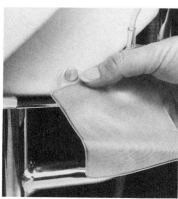

11 Attach the collection bag to the hanger at the pump case's right corner. To call up the next screen, press ENTER.

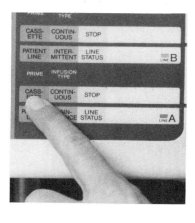

12 The display screen now says: *HOLD DOWN [CASSETTE] KEY ON A TO PRIME INTO COLLECTION BAG. PRESS [ENTER].* Locate the CASSETTE key for Line A, and hold down this key to prime the primary line. Press ENTER when you see solution flow into the collection bag.

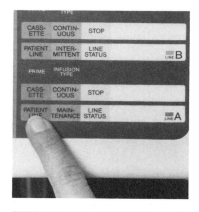

13 To prime the patient line, press PATIENT LINE on Line A's line status panel.

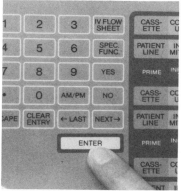

14 When all the air clears, press ENTER. Note the display screen, which says: *CASSETTE TEST IN PROGRESS.*

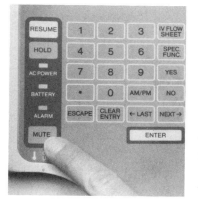

15 If this 36-second test identifies a problem, the pump sounds an alarm and the display screen reads: *POSSIBLE FAULTY CASSETTE/REPRIME OR REPLACE CASSETTE.* Press the MUTE key twice to silence the alarm, then reprime the cassette. If the alarm sounds again, replace the cassette. If you continue to have problems, send the pump out for servicing.

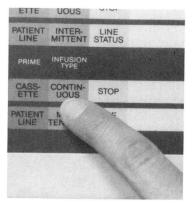

16 If the pump checks out, however, the display screen reads: *SELECT LINE INFUSION TYPE/PRESS [CONTINUOUS] OR [INTERMITTENT].* Enter the ordered infusion type (mode). Now you're ready to prime the secondary lines (see following photostory).

Priming an Omni-Flow secondary line

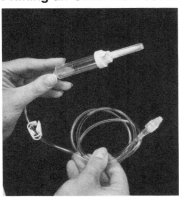

1 Follow this procedure to prime each secondary line. Remove the secondary set from the package and close the clamp.

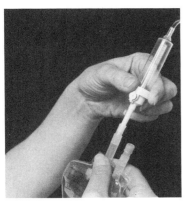

2 Obtain the ordered I.V. solution. Check its label, noting medication, dose, and preparation date. Spike the container and hang it on the pole.

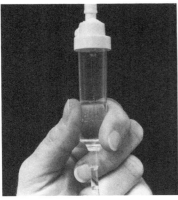

3 Squeeze the drip chamber to set the fluid level. Open the clamp and clear air from the I.V. line.

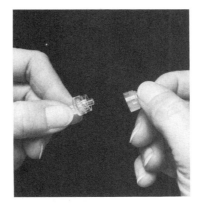

4 Close the clamp and remove the Luer-Lok protector from the secondary set.

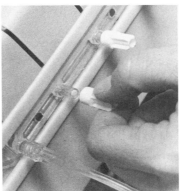

5 Next, remove the Luer-Lok protector on Line B's cassette connector, as shown.

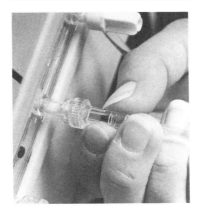

6 Connect the secondary set to the cassette, open the clamp, and check to see that no fluid flows into the drip chamber.
Repeat the procedure to prime additional lines.

Connecting a syringe to the cassette

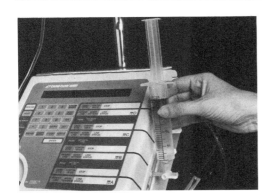

You can use a syringe to infuse medication through the cassette. To attach the syringe to the cassette, remove the Luer-Lok protector on one of the cassette's secondary line connectors. Connect a three-way stopcock to the connector.

Then, connect a 10-ml (or larger) syringe of medication to the stopcock so that the syringe points up, as shown here. Turn the stopcock to open a pathway between the syringe and the cassette. After you program the infusion mode, the pump will draw medication from the syringe by suction.

I.V. therapy

Programming the primary line

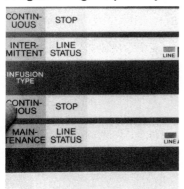

1 If you want the primary line (Line A) to infuse continuously, even when other lines inject intermittent doses, choose the continuous mode. If you want the primary infusion to stop during intermittent doses, choose the maintenance mode.

To program the primary line for a continuous infusion, press Line A's CONTINUOUS key, as shown. Then press ENTER.

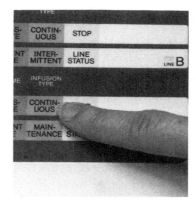

5 If you want to make a rate change after the infusion starts, just depress the CONTINUOUS key, enter the change, and press ENTER.

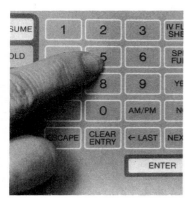

2 Input the ordered rate per hour, using the numerical keyboard. The display screen shows you the rate you've entered. Press ENTER.

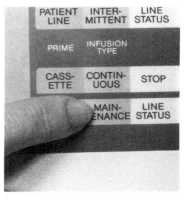

6 To program the primary line in the maintenance mode, press the MAINTENANCE key for Line A, as shown.

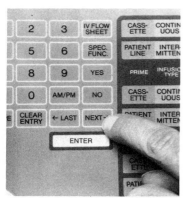

3 Press the NEXT key to move the cursor. Then input the total volume to be infused. The screen shows you the volume you've entered.

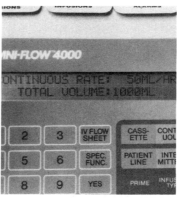

7 Set the rate and volume (see Steps 2 and 3). The display screen shows the values you've entered (see photo). Press ENTER to start the infusion.

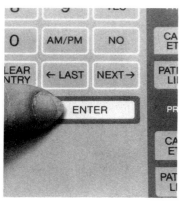

4 Press ENTER to start the infusion. The display screen reports on each line.

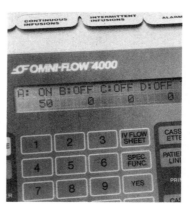

8 The display screen now shows Line A's status, as shown here.

Stopping infusions and removing the cassette

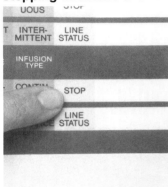

1 Press the STOP key on each line's line function panel. Press ENTER.

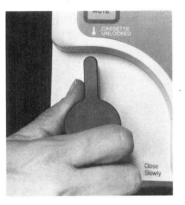

2 To remove the cassette, make sure the pump is switched on and all lines are off. Then close the clamps and remove the collection bag from the holder.
   Lift the cassette locking lever toward you and turn it counter-clockwise.

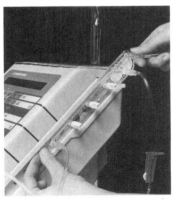

3 Slide the cassette out of the holder.

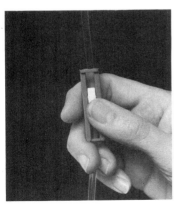

4 Using the roller clamp, regulate the primary I.V. line at the ordered I.V. rate.

Programming secondary lines for intermittent infusions

You can program a secondary line to deliver intermittent infusions for up to 24 hours. To do so, press the INTERMITTENT key on whichever line you want to use. Then, following the display screen's instructions, enter this information:
- volume to be infused
- time for each infusion (the pump automatically calculates rate)
- infusion frequency (hours between doses)
- number of infusions.
   If you wish, you can program such additional functions as:
- setting call-back alarm
- administering an infusion from a syringe
- diluting an infusion with solution from the primary line.
   Note: The pump will infuse only one intermittent dose at a time. If you inadvertently schedule two at the same time, the pump infuses them in alphabetical order: line B, then C, then D.

How the Vena-Vue Vein Evaluator reveals hard-to-find veins

Even if you're highly skilled at venipuncture, you're occasionally stymied by a patient with hard-to-find veins. A new tool, the Vena-Vue Vein Evaluator, could save such a patient the discomfort of several futile venipuncture attempts.
   A thin elastic thermographic film, Vena-Vue delineates patent veins by changing color when you apply it over a likely venipuncture site and cool it with ice. A patent vein rewarms faster than surrounding tissue. Liquid crystals in the Vena-Vue strip respond to this warmth with a well-delineated color pattern. You then mark the vein with a special probe (supplied by the manufacturer), remove the film, and proceed with venipuncture.

Using Vena-Vue

Follow this procedure:
- Select a promising venipuncture site—preferably on the hand or forearm. Don't apply a tourniquet.
- Apply the film to the skin, pressing firmly to ensure adhesion.
- Remove the film's protective backing.
- Note the film's color. A uniform black color indicates good peripheral circulation. However, if you see a diffuse color pattern (tan, green, blue, and violet), consider peripheral circulation poor.

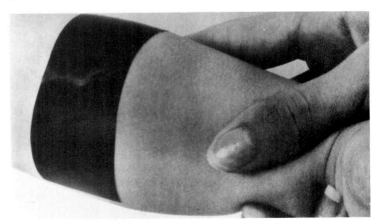

Color changes on the Vena-Vue film delineate a patent vein.

I.V. therapy

How the Vena-Vue Vein Evaluator reveals hard-to-find veins
continued

• Take steps to dilate the veins—for example, by applying compresses, immersing the site in warm water, or asking the patient to clench and unclench his fist.
• Use ice to cool the film and surrounding skin evenly on either side. Watch the film change colors, from black to violet, blue, green, and tan. *Note:* Don't overcool.
• Hold the arm at heart level.
• Wait about 2 minutes for a pattern to develop. *Note:* If color changes don't occur after cooling and rewarming, the underlying vein isn't patent. Select an alternative site.
• Press the probe against the film over the vein. The probe leaves a temporary skin depression that will guide you during venipuncture. Mark proximal and distal portions of the delineated vein on the film. (Use the probe on your own arm first to feel how much pressure you need to leave a skin mark.)
• Remove the film from the patient's skin. Prepare the skin, apply a tourniquet if you wish, and proceed with venipuncture.

Interpreting a Vena-Vue pattern
Variations in the Vena-Vue color pattern give you additional information about the target vein. For example:
• a parallel pattern that develops evenly across the film indicates a patent vein directly underneath.
• a comet pattern indicates a descending vein that's closest to the skin at the pattern's widest point.
• an elliptical pattern indicates an arched vein that's closest to the surface at the pattern's widest point.
• a diffuse pattern indicates occluded or sclerosed veins.

Venipuncture sites in the antecubital fossa

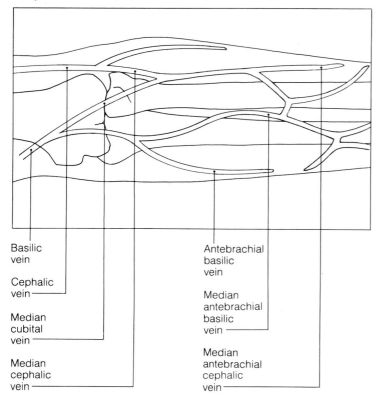

Basilic vein

Cephalic vein

Median cubital vein

Median cephalic vein

Antebrachial basilic vein

Median antebrachial basilic vein

Median antebrachial cephalic vein

The CRIS system: A new way to deliver secondary I.V. drugs
If you've ever wished for an easy and cost-effective way to administer secondary drugs through a primary I.V. line, take a look at IVAC's Controlled Release Infusion System (CRIS). Connected to the I.V. line between the primary container and the administration set, the CRIS adapter lets you administer a drug dose without using a minibag and piggyback administration set. You simply attach a single-dose vial to the CRIS spike and turn the CRIS valve handle toward the vial (as shown in the following photostory). The primary infusion flows into the vial and mixes with the drug; the mixture then flows down the line to the patient. You can use the CRIS system with any I.V. solution container, any primary set, and either instrumented or noninstrumented lines.

Besides simplicity, the CRIS system has these benefits that can increase your productivity:
• You needn't interrupt the primary flow to administer a secondary drug.
• You don't have to flush tubing between drugs.
• Because you use only one solution container, you can monitor fluid intake more easily.
• The system saves the time you'd ordinarily spend priming secondary sets, adjusting and readjusting primary and secondary flow rates, and handling secondary containers.
• The system also saves the storage space you'd need for minibags and secondary I.V. sets.

Use the CRIS adapter with unvented I.V. tubing and reconstituted drugs in single-dose vials (from 5 to 20 ml). *Important:* For safe, effective use, read and follow the manufacturer's recommendations.

CRIS adapter

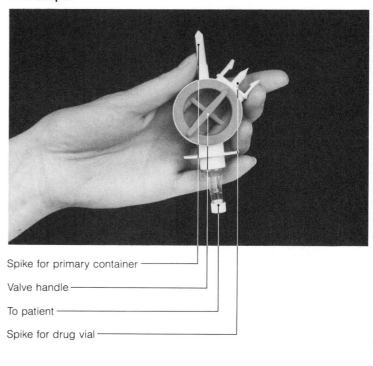

Spike for primary container

Valve handle

To patient

Spike for drug vial

How to use a CRIS adapter

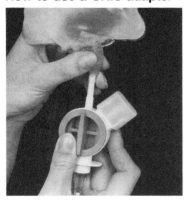

1 Install the CRIS adapter on the patient's I.V. line. (*Push* the administration set's spike into the CRIS' lower port—don't twist.) Obtain a single-dose vial of reconstituted drug (as ordered) and an alcohol swab.

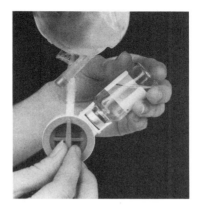

5 Before giving another drug dose, make sure the primary I.V. container holds at least 60 ml fluid. Then turn the valve handle to the 12 o'clock position.

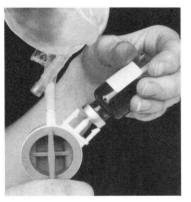

2 Remove the vial's temporary cover and clean its diaphragm with the swab. Using a twisting motion, remove the CRIS vial spike's protective cover and impale the vial on the spike. ✆*Nursing tip:* If you encounter resistance, puncture the diaphragm with a needle to release air.

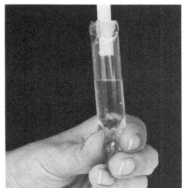

6 Adjust the drip chamber's fluid level, if necessary. (Don't squeeze the drip chamber during drug administration, or you may force the drug into the primary container.)

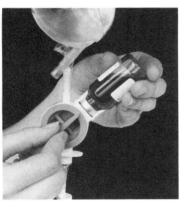

3 Make sure the primary container holds at least 60 ml fluid—the volume needed to deliver the dose and flush the system. Then, to begin drug delivery, turn the valve handle toward the vial until you feel resistance. Click the valve into place in the 2 o'clock position.
Calculate the flow rate and set the pump appropriately. (Or mark the container or time tape.)

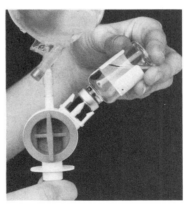

7 Remove the used vial and replace it with the new one, as described earlier.

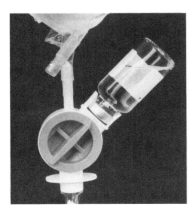

4 After drug delivery's complete, leave the vial in place and keep the valve handle in the 2 o'clock position until you're ready to deliver another drug dose. (Note that because the primary infusion flows through the vial, the vial doesn't empty.) Leaving the vial in place maintains the vial spike's sterility.

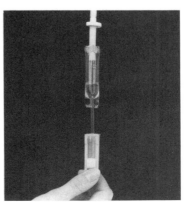

8 Turn the valve handle back to the 2 o'clock position. Adjust the flow rate.
Change the CRIS adapter when you change the administration set—every 48 hours or according to hospital policy. *Note:* You can use the CRIS adapter on a primary line while delivering another drug through a piggyback set.

I.V. therapy

Using a multiple-lumen catheter

Here's the scenario: You've got a patient who's already receiving intermittent I.V. antibiotics and a continuous heparin infusion through separate I.V. lines. Now you have to prepare him for I.V. hyperalimentation (IVH). In the past, this would have meant a third I.V. site—and a growing risk of infection and other complications.

If you've ever wished for a simpler system, you now have it: multiple-lumen central venous catheters can deliver several infusions simultaneously through two, three, or four separate lumens contained in the same I.V. line.

Lumen sizes vary, so the catheter can accommodate such viscous liquids as blood and IVH solutions, as well as drugs and I.V. fluids. Its distal lumen provides central venous pressure measurements. Because it's so versatile, it may be ordered for a variety of patients, including burn, trauma, and heart attack victims; surgical, oncologic, and long-term intensive care unit patients; and patients who are dehydrated or malnourished. Contraindications include recurrent sepsis and heparin sensitivity.

Insertion: Your role
If you're assisting with catheter insertion, take the usual preliminary steps: explain the procedure to the patient and his family, check for allergies, and make sure the patient has signed a consent form, if required by hospital policy. Also obtain the equipment and establish a sterile field. Then:
• place the patient in Trendelenburg's posi-

tion (unless contraindicated) to dilate veins and reduce the risk of air embolism.
• put a rolled towel lengthwise between his shoulders if the doctor plans a subclavian insertion: this helps distend the vein. For jugular insertion, place a rolled towel under the shoulder opposite the insertion site.
• turn the patient's head away from the insertion site to minimize contamination risks. (The doctor may ask you to mask the patient to further minimize risks.)
• make sure an X-ray confirms proper placement.
• document catheter placement, the insertion site, central venous pressure, and the patient's response to the procedure. Label the dressing with the time and date of catheter insertion and with the catheter length (if not imprinted on the catheter). Also label each lumen to show what's being infused through it.

Catheter care: Special considerations
During therapy, take the same measures you'd use to care for any central venous catheter. In addition, remember these points:
• Clamp the catheter before opening any lumen to air.
• If you're not using all of the catheter lumens, cover each unused port with a heparin lock cap and flush each lumen with 100 units of heparin every 6 to 12 hours (according to hospital policy). Also flush each lumen after intermittent use.
• When heparinizing, clamp the catheter when you're infusing the last 0.5 ml, to create

positive pressure and prevent clotting.
• Disinfect the adapter for 2 minutes before any injection. Also disinfect the connection between the intermittent infusion device adapter and the lumen for 2 minutes before disconnection.
• Change Luer-Lok intermittent injection caps every 3 days. (Clamp the catheter first.)
• Use only 20G 1″ needles to puncture a Luer-Lok injection cap.
• To prevent a bulky four-lumen catheter from twisting, tape the four lumens to a padded tongue blade.

Complications
Any central venous catheter can cause complications, such as infection, heart perforation, pneumothorax, and air embolism. The catheter itself may become occluded or break from excessive force or overuse.

Throughout therapy, monitor the patient closely for signs and symptoms of pneumothorax (shortness of breath, tachycardia, and/or chest pain) and air embolism (pallor, cyanosis, dyspnea, coughing, tachycardia, syncope, and/or shock). Notify the doctor immediately if any of these signs or symptoms occur. If you suspect air embolism, turn the patient on his left side in Trendelenburg's position.

If the patient develops an infection, the doctor may attempt to treat it by administering antibiotics through the catheter. Or he may remove the catheter. He may clear an occlusion by injecting urokinase into the blocked lumen.

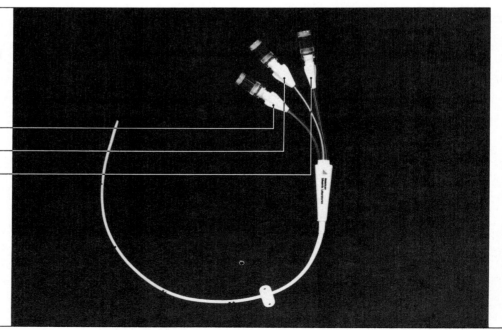

This triple-lumen Multi-Med Infusion Catheter (American Edwards Laboratories) has a heparin coating to help prevent thrombus formation. Like all such catheters, it has color-coded lumen ports.

2 cm proximal lumen port (18 gauge) ——————

Distal lumen port (16 gauge) ——————

5 cm proximal lumen port (18 gauge) ——————

Postoperative care

When you care for a postoperative patient, you must anticipate a variety of potential problems, including infection and immobility complications. In this section, we'll acquaint you with new tools that make your job easier and improve patient care.

To help you monitor the patient's temperature, you may use a device like the Mon-a-therm continuous temperature monitor, which provides continuous temperature information on up to three body sites simultaneously. A simpler system, the digital temperature detector, lets you estimate body temperature at a glance.

If your patient faces a period of immobility, he's at risk for such problems as loss of joint movement, deep vein thrombosis, and pressure sores. The following equipment helps you minimize immobility hazards:

• Mediscus Air Support Therapy System, a unique bed that supports the patient on air sacs inflated to therapeutic pressures that best suit his height, weight, and body distribution

• Danniflex Continuous Passive Motion System, which provides passive joint exercise after orthopedic surgery

• T.E.D. Sequential Compression Device, which helps maintain blood flow velocity in the legs, thus guarding against deep vein thrombosis.

We'll also feature an easy-to-use chest tube drainage system, a handy suture-removal tool, and pads designed to prevent or treat pressure sores at bony prominences.

Continuous temperature monitoring: Combining precision with versatility

During and after surgery, your patient may need precise, continuous temperature monitoring to detect hyperthermia or hypothermia. A system such as the Mon-a-therm Model 7000 Temperature Monitoring System (see photo) can help you provide the best possible care.

The Mon-a-therm Model 7000, a lightweight, microprocessor-based digital display monitor, permits continuous assessment of body temperature at one to three sites, with an accuracy of ±0.1° C. or ±0.2° F. Disposable sensors placed at various body sites provide the monitor with temperature input. For example, a urinary bladder catheter sensor accurately provides core body temperature readings.

Besides continuous temperature display, the Mon-a-therm Model 7000 provides visual and audible alarm systems for each display, with adjustable alarm set switches; an elapsed time display; and a 2-hour temperature trend indicator that can recall the previous 6 hours for Site 1 as well as the temperature difference between Sites 1 and 2. And the system has computer interface capability, a built-in calibration check feature, and a battery replacement indicator.

Read the photostory beginning on page 88 for details on how to set up and operate this system.

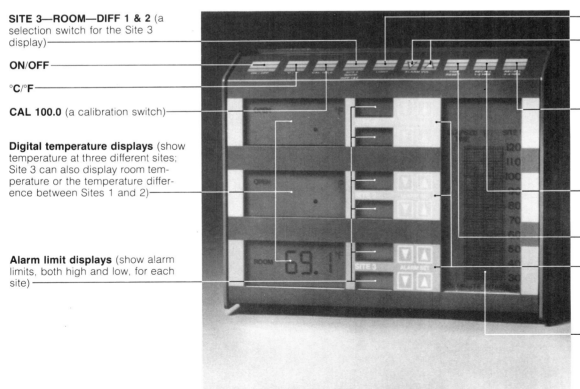

SITE 3—ROOM—DIFF 1 & 2 (a selection switch for the Site 3 display)

ON/OFF

°C/°F

CAL 100.0 (a calibration switch)

Digital temperature displays (show temperature at three different sites; Site 3 can also display room temperature or the temperature difference between Sites 1 and 2)

Alarm limit displays (show alarm limits, both high and low, for each site)

LIGHT

ALARM VOL (increases or decreases alarm volume; silences alarm when both increase and decrease buttons are pressed simultaneously)

RECALL 3-4 HRS (recalls the 3rd and 4th hours of temperature history after the timer starts. To recall the 5th and 6th hours, simultaneously press RECALL 1-2 HRS and RECALL 3-4 HRS.)

RECALL 1-2 HRS (recalls the first 2 hours of temperature history after the timer starts)

TIME RESET (starts the timer and resets the history display)

ALARM SET switches (increase or decrease alarm limits for each site; separate audio and visual alarms beep and flash when alarm limits are exceeded)

Temperature trend display (shows temperature trend for 2 hours graphically, with recall of 6 hours using the RECALL switches)

Postoperative care

Learning about disposable sensors

When you use a system such as the Mon-a-therm Model 7000, you need to be familiar with the variety of sensors that provide the monitor with information. Depending on your patient's condition and on the doctor's preference, any of these disposable sensors may provide input for the Mon-a-therm 7000's temperature displays. (The manufacturer also offers subcutaneous and thermal well sensors.)

Myocardial sensor
Useful during hypothermic cardio-plegia; available in 8-, 18-, and 38-mm sizes

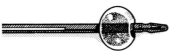

Urinary bladder catheter sensor
Provides body core temperature correlating to pulmonary artery blood temperature in any patient needing an indwelling catheter; available in 10, 12, 16, or 18 French

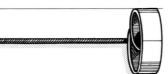

Digit temperature sensor
Measures extremity temperature (usually applied to the big toe)

Skin sensor
Adheres to skin and responds rapidly to skin temperature changes

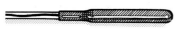

Esophageal stethoscope with temperature sensor
Monitors heart, lung, and breath sounds while sensing temperature; available in 9, 12, 18, or 24 French

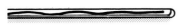

Esophageal/rectal sensor
Monitors esophageal or rectal temperature

Tympanic sensor
Provides true core body temperature, offering an alternative to an esophageal sensor

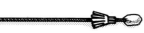

Luer-Lok sensor
Measures the temperature of fluids or gases at the site of any Luer-Lok connection

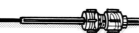

Nasopharyngeal sensor
Measures temperature in the post-nasal space

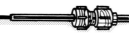

Airway sensor
Detects airway temperature changes (adapts to most breathing circuits); available in adult and pediatric sizes

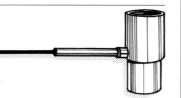

Operating the Mon-a-therm Model 7000 Temperature Monitoring System

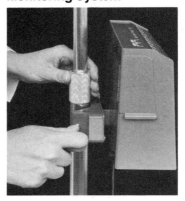

1 Mount the Mon-a-therm 7000 on an I.V. pole and position it so that you can easily view the front. You may tilt the instrument once it's mounted to provide the best viewing angle.

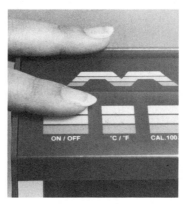

2 Press the ON/OFF switch to turn the monitor on, as shown. You'll hear a beep; then all display areas will light, showing 188.8 at each temperature display site and at all six of the alarm display sites. All the annunciators will light, and the temperature trend scale will be completely filled in.

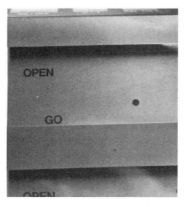

3 The instrument will complete a self-checking procedure. If everything's functioning correctly, it will display *GO* for about 6 seconds at each display site. (If it finds an electronic problem, it will display *NO GO* at one or more sites; in that case, contact a service representative and don't use the monitor.)

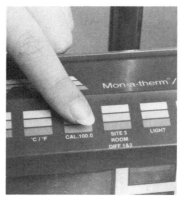

4 Press and hold down the CAL. 100.0 switch. Check the three temperature displays—they should show 100 ± 0.3. (If they don't, return the monitor for calibration.)

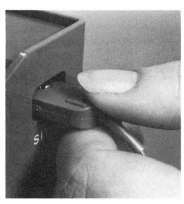

5 For each site you're planning to use, connect a sensor cable to the appropriate receptacle on the instrument's side, as shown. (Place unused storage cables in the cable storage compartment on the instrument's opposite side.) Make sure you insert the cable into the receptacle right-side up—instrument damage or false readings can result from forcing the cable connectors in upside down.

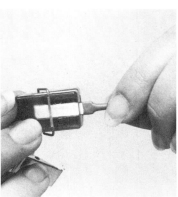

6 Connect a temperature sensor to each sensor cable, as ordered. Open the cable connector completely, pressing on the toggle's back portion with your thumb. Insert the sensor's flat rectangular end— with the contacts up—into the open connector, making sure you position the rectangular end against the connector's rear wall. Check correct placement by looking through the connector's clear base.

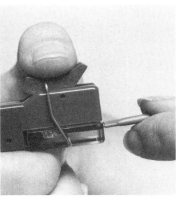

7 Secure the connection by pressing the front part of the toggle with your thumb. Then, to prevent strain on the temperature sensor wire, fasten the alligator clip (located near the cable connector) to the patient's gown or drape.

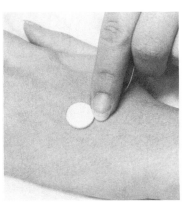

8 After explaining the procedure to the patient, apply or insert the appropriate sensors, as ordered, or assist the doctor, as required. For example, you might apply a skin sensor for Site 1 (as shown), insert a urinary bladder sensor (CathTemp) for Site 2, and leave Site 3 open to measure the temperature difference between Sites 1 and 2.

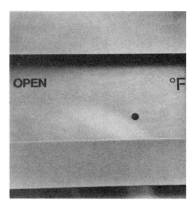

9 Check the temperature displays. If you haven't connected a sensor to a site, or if you've connected a defective sensor, you'll see *OPEN* in the display's upper left corner, as shown here. However, if a sensor you've connected to a site functions properly, the display shows the patient's temperature. Depress the °C/°F switch to adjust the display for Celsius or Fahrenheit.

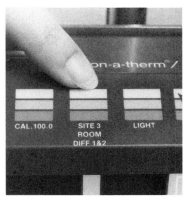

10 The Site 3 display shows room temperature initially. If you want it to display Site 3 temperature or the difference between Sites 1 and 2, press the SITE 3—ROOM—DIFF 1 & 2 switch, which will move the display successively through the three modes. (For example, if you press the switch while the display shows ROOM, it advances to DIFF 1 & 2 and shows the temperature difference between Sites 1 and 2.)

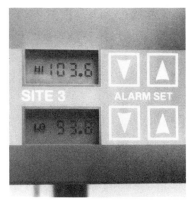

11 Each ALARM SET display has high and low indicator buttons marked with arrows. On initial use, or after new battery insertion, the alarms come on at their extreme low and high settings; otherwise, they come on at the values they were set to when the instrument was last used. Change the set point rapidly by pressing continuously on the appropriate arrow; make fine adjustments by pushing the arrow briefly.

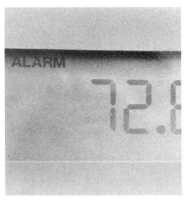

12 When measured temperature exceeds one of the set points, a beep will sound, the display will flash, and *ALARM* will appear on the appropriate display. *Note:* You can disable the alarm by changing the set point to a temperature at which the site's no longer in an alarm condition.

Postoperative care

Operating the Mon-a-therm Model 7000 Temperature Monitoring System continued

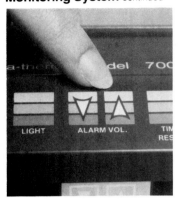

13 Adjust the audible alarm with the two arrows at the instrument's top. To shut off the audible alarm, press both arrows simultaneously. (*Note:* Shutting off the audible alarm won't affect the visual ALARM display or stop the display from blinking.)

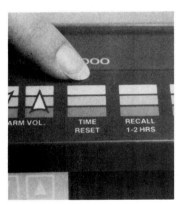

14 To use the temperature trend display, press the TIME RESET switch. A graph of Site 1 temperature over time will appear, unless Site 3 is in DIFF mode. If you see DIFF at the graph's upper right, the graph will display a history of the temperature difference between Sites 1 and 2.

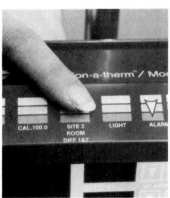

15 To select the Site 1 temperature trend display when the instrument's in DIFF mode, push the SITE 3—ROOM—DIFF 1 & 2 switch. The graph will immediately display a dot at its far left edge, representing Site 1 temperature in ° F. or ° C., as selected. A new dot will appear to the right of the previous one every 15 minutes; after the first 2 hours, one dot disappears from the left side for each dot added to the right side.

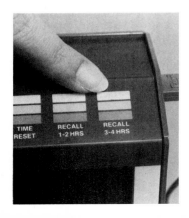

16 To recall temperature history information for the first 6 hours after you pressed TIME RESET, press RECALL 1-2 HRS, RECALL 3-4 HRS, or both at once (to display information for the 5th and 6th hours). *Note:* If the monitor's accidentally switched off, the temperature history information stored in memory won't be lost if you turn the instrument back on within 15 seconds.

Adhesive temperature detectors: Convenient and noninvasive

After surgery, you need to monitor your patient's temperature frequently. You can do so at a glance with the Stat-Temp temperature detector, a small disk with a metal substrate backing and a hypoallergenic adhesive. After you apply it to the patient's forehead, a liquid crystal continuously shows a digital reading reflecting body core temperature. A correction factor converts skin temperature to estimated oral temperature.

Stat-Temp has a range of 95° to 107° F., or 35° to 41.7° C. (A wider-range model, Stat-Temp WR, detects temperatures ranging from 82° to 107° F., or 27.8° to 41.7° C.) Because sebaceous secretions degrade its adhesive, Stat-Temp remains accurate for only about 24 hours (and shorter periods when applied to a diaphoretic patient).

Here's how to use Stat-Temp:

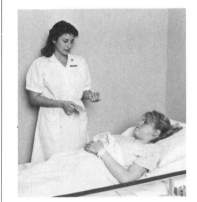

1 Show your patient the detector. Tell her you're going to stick it to her forehead so you can monitor her temperature without a probe or thermometer.

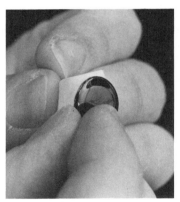

2 Remove the protective backing and apply the detector to her forehead, as shown in Step 3. Because the correction factor's specific for the indicated site (the forehead, close to the hairline), make sure you position the detector correctly.

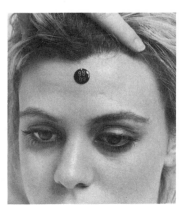

3 Wait a few seconds, then read the results (indoors at room temperature, away from a cold breeze or direct sunlight). If two numbers show clearly, the correct reading's in between them (ignore numbers in blue). For example, read 99° F. if you see both 98° and 100° F. Estimate temperature between digital steps by interpreting the displayed digits' color, which can range from violet at the coolest limit of visibility to green at the warmest.

Using Thora-Drain III

Jane Hall, a 39-year-old secretary, enters your unit with minor injuries sustained in an auto accident. The next day, she develops a hemothorax. While the doctor inserts a chest tube, you prepare to connect the tube to a Thora-Drain III Underwater Drainage System, a closed-chest, water-seal drainage system.

You'll recall that water-seal drainage uses water to create a seal, or one-way valve, which allows accumulated fluid to leave the pleural space and prevents it from reentering. Removing excess fluid and air permits the pleural cavity to regain negative pressure, which allows the lungs to reexpand.

A three-chamber unit with connecting tubing, Thora-Drain III provides drainage collection, a water seal, and suction control. Compared to similar disposable units, it has a unique feature: a replaceable collection compartment. When the compartment fills, you replace it; however, you don't replace the rest of the unit.

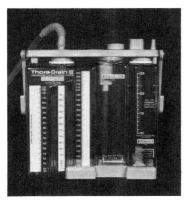

1 To set up the system, assemble this equipment: a Thora-Drain III Underwater Drainage System (shown here), sterile normal saline solution, a suction device, and 1" tape.

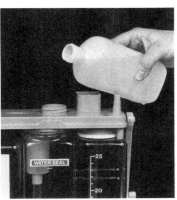

2 Using aseptic technique, remove the water-seal chamber's cap and pour about 120 ml of normal saline solution into the chamber until the solution level reaches the indicator line. Replace the cap securely. *Note:* To ensure an effective seal, maintain this fluid level. Check the chamber frequently and refill when necessary.

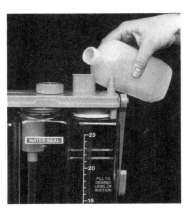

3 Now, fill the suction-control chamber with normal saline solution to the ordered suction level.

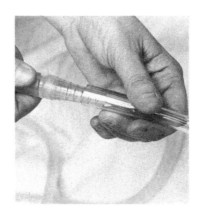

4 You're now ready to connect the chest tube to the drainage unit. Explain the procedure to the patient. Then remove the connecting tubing's blue cover and attach the tubing to the patient's chest tube, as shown.

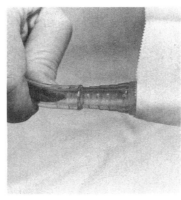

5 Tape the tube securely above and below the connector. You've now established water-seal drainage. Check to see that the connecting tubing remains on the bed. Don't let loops form.

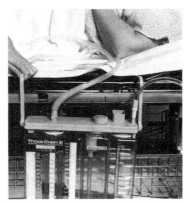

6 Next, secure the Thora-Drain III unit to the patient's bed, using the attached hooks, as shown. Make sure the unit remains as far below the patient's chest as possible. *Note:* If the unit tips over, set it upright immediately. The system prevents fluid from spilling or mixing with fluid in other chambers.

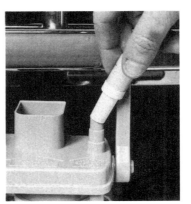

7 Finally, attach the suction device tubing to the suction port. After you turn on the suction, you should see gentle bubbling in the suction-control chamber.

Postoperative care

Thora-Drain III: Special considerations

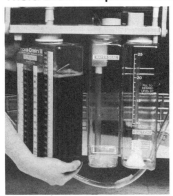

1 When your patient's drainage chamber fills up, follow these steps to replace it. Obtain a Thora-Drain III replacement chamber and remove it from its sterile package. *Note:* If hospital policy requires it, double-clamp the chest tube close to the insertion site before replacing the chamber.

Then twist the collection chamber to the left to loosen it, as shown. Remove the chamber.

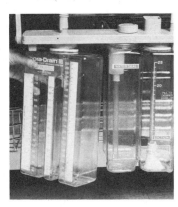

2 Remove the replacement chamber's cap. Position the chamber as shown, and turn it to the left; then lock it in place by turning it to the right. (If you clamped the chest tube, remove the clamps now.)

Then replace the filled collection chamber's cap. Note the drainage amount, color, and consistency before discarding it, and document your findings.

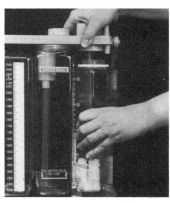

3 To reduce the suction level, first discontinue the suction. Then remove the suction chamber, rotating it to the left.

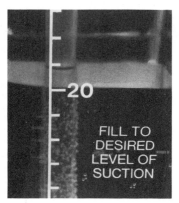

4 Adjust the fluid level and replace the chamber, snapping it in place to the right. Reconnect the suction.

Closed-chest drainage: Points to remember

Use this checklist when caring for a patient with any closed-chest drainage system.

Assessing and teaching the patient
• Evaluate the patient's condition frequently. Report any changes, including rapid, shallow breathing; subcutaneous emphysema; excessive drainage; cyanosis; or chest pain.
• Teach him about his chest drainage system. Instruct him to report any disconnections immediately and to keep the drainage unit below chest level.

Checking chest and drainage tubing
• Check the chest tube connection for signs of an air leak, such as a hissing sound. Check the tube frequently for tears, punctures, and other damage affecting its integrity.
• Make sure the chest tube dressing remains secure.
• Keep the drainage tubing on the patient's bed. Don't permit dependent loops and kinks to form.

Observing the collection chamber
• Every hour, record drainage volume and character. Report increased or decreased volume. Consider more than 100 ml/hour excessive. If drainage stops, check for an obstruction.
• When the collection chamber fills, replace the compartment or unit according to the manufacturer's instructions.

Maintaining a water seal
• Listen for hissing sounds, which indicate an air leak.
• Turn off suction control briefly and observe for tidaling: fluctuations in the water-seal chamber as the patient breathes, indicating an intact water seal. If you don't see tidaling, check the tube for patency and report the problem. *Note:* Tidaling stops when the lung reexpands. Also, you won't see it if the patient has a mediastinal chest tube.
• Check for bubbling, which could indicate an air leak. *Note:* Expect to see bubbling if the patient has a pneumothorax; bubbling decreases as his lung reexpands.
• Keep the water-seal chamber filled at all times to ensure negative pressure.

Checking suction control
• Maintain the ordered suction pressure.
• Expect to see gentle bubbling in this chamber. The doctor may reduce suction if bubbling becomes excessive.

Learning about continuous passive motion devices

Lucy Reichert, a tennis pro, just had surgery to repair torn knee ligaments. A few years ago, she'd have been ordered to lie motionless in bed for a week or more. But now her orthopedic surgeon says that motion—not immobilization—will speed recovery and maybe even save Ms. Reichert's athletic career. Consequently, you have the responsibility for setting up a new piece of equipment: a continuous passive motion (CPM) device that will move her knee without putting weight on the joint or tiring the muscles.

Studies show that CPM stimulates the healing and regeneration of articular tissues and prevents or minimizes joint stiffness. The doctor may order it following a variety of procedures, including total joint replacement, reconstruction of ligaments, internal fixation of fractures, arthrotomy for posttraumatic arthritis, and other orthopedic procedures.

The device shown below, the Danniflex 400SL Continuous Passive Motion System (Danninger Medical), keeps an orthopedic patient's hip, knee, and ankle moving. It works like the driving rods on the sides of a steam locomotive, cyclically drawing the leg up at the knee and then extending it in one fluid motion. You can set the CPM device's speed and degree of flexion and extension. A control cord allows the patient to stop or start the device as

desired. Other CPM devices provide motion to injured shoulders, elbows, and hands.

Precautions and troubleshooting tips
Learn to set up the Danniflex 400SL CPM system by reading the following photostories. When you're ready to use it, remember these points.

Make sure that the coiled cord from the drive unit base to the goniometer hangs freely. If you move the unit, don't stretch the cord. Also, don't operate the equipment near flammable gases.

If you have trouble operating the unit, check:
• the red power light. If it doesn't come on when you turn on the power, check to see if the unit's properly plugged into an outlet. Also check the circuit breaker on the controller's rear panel.
• the patient control cord. If the unit doesn't respond to commands given through the cord, make sure the cord is firmly attached to the controller. If it is, and the unit works without it, replace the cord.
• the FLEXION and EXTENSION dials. The unit won't work if they're set within 5 degrees of each other or if the EXTENSION setting is higher then the FLEXION setting.

Danniflex 400SL drive unit orthosis

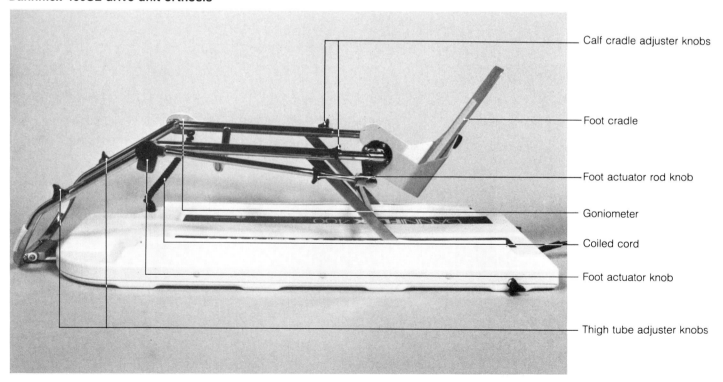

Calf cradle adjuster knobs
Foot cradle
Foot actuator rod knob
Goniometer
Coiled cord
Foot actuator knob
Thigh tube adjuster knobs

Postoperative care

How to set up the Danniflex 400SL CPM System

Before you begin, unpack the equipment and make sure you have the drive unit orthosis (shown on the previous page), the electronic controller (shown below), and these other components: patient control cord, kit containing pads, and thigh shield. (An assembly for mounting the drive unit orthosis on the bed is also included.)
Important: *Check the serial numbers on the drive unit orthosis and the controller—the last four digits should be identical.*

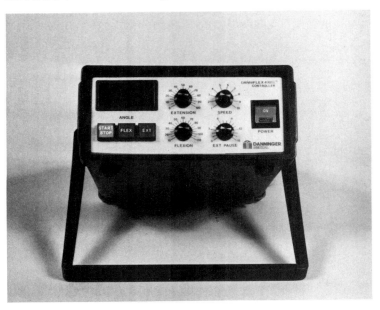

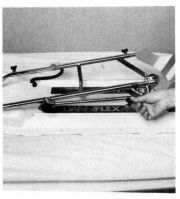

1 Screw the foot actuator rod knob into the small outer rod connected to the foot cradle. Don't tighten the knob.

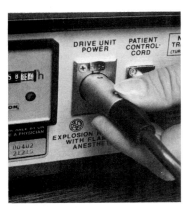

2 Plug the power cable (located behind the foot cradle) into the large receptacle on the controller's back. Align the pins and push the plug gently into place.

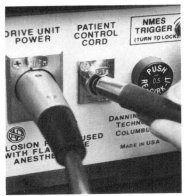

3 Attach the patient control cord to the other receptacle on the controller's back. (Use the cord's clip to attach the cord to the bedcovers, if you wish.)

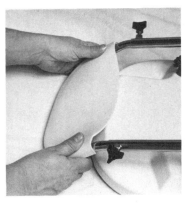

4 Attach the Velcro-backed thigh shield to the unit by pressing it in place, as shown.

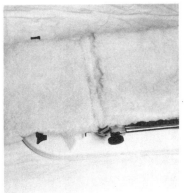

5 Take the pads from the kit. Place the rounded pad on the thigh section and secure it with its Velcro-backed straps.
Then attach the rectangular covering to the calf cradle in the same manner. Make sure the narrow strap passes directly behind the goniometer. (Don't wrap straps around the foot actuator rod.)

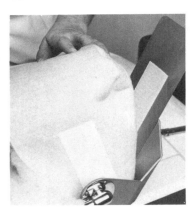

6 Finally, attach the boot to the foot cradle. The boot's sole adheres to the foot cradle.

Positioning the patient

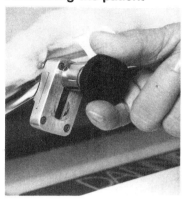

1 After you set up the Danni-flex 400SL CPM system, adjust the unit to fit your patient. First, set the foot actuator in neutral (the highest position) and tighten the foot actuator knob, as shown.

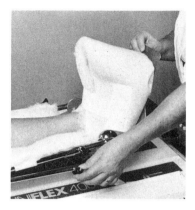

5 How you adjust the foot assembly depends on the exercises the doctor orders. To keep the foot and ankle motionless, leave the foot actuator in neutral (highest) position and set the foot cradle at the ordered angle. Then tighten the foot actuator rod knob, as shown.

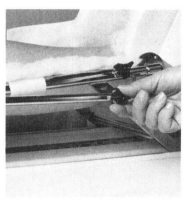

2 Then unscrew the foot actuator rod knob, as shown. The foot actuator can now move freely during the adjustment process.

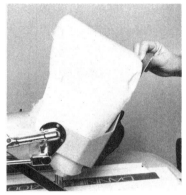

6 For full flexion of the foot and ankle, loosen the foot actuator rod knob and allow the foot cradle to drop to its lowest point.

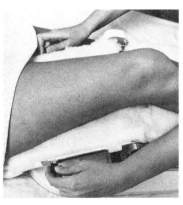

3 After measuring the length of the patient's thigh (gluteal crease to knee), loosen the adjuster knobs on both thigh tubes. Lengthen or shorten the thigh tubes to fit thigh length, and tighten the adjuster knobs.

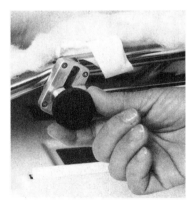

7 Then loosen the foot actuator knob (as shown), set it at the lowest position, and tighten it securely. (For partial ankle flexion, set the foot actuator knob at any point between the highest and lowest position.) Then raise the foot cradle about ¼″ and tighten the foot actuator rod knob.

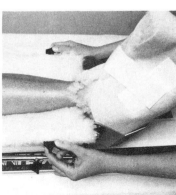

4 Similarly, measure the length of the patient's lower leg (knee to heel). Loosen the adjustment knobs on each side of the calf cradle. Lengthen or shorten, as needed, and tighten the adjuster knobs, as shown.

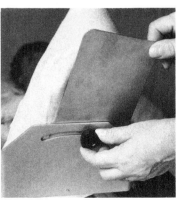

8 For foot rotation, loosen the adjuster knob at the foot cradle's back and reset it to the right or left, as needed.
Note: If you readjust the calf cradle, remember to temporarily loosen the foot actuator rod knob. Readjust both sides, or you may damage the unit.

Postoperative care

Operating the Danniflex 400SL controller

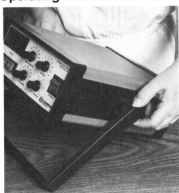

1 Set the controller on a level surface. Prop it on its handle to position the control panel conveniently. Press the handle rotation buttons to allow the handle to move freely.

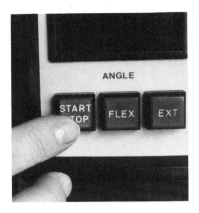

5 Press the START/STOP button. The controller automatically initiates action, beginning with extension. (To reverse direction manually, use the FLEX and EXT buttons.)

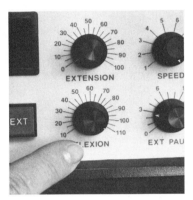

2 Turn the extension dial to the lowest reading and the flexion dial to the highest reading. Turn on the power.

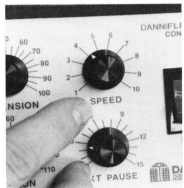

6 Set the SPEED dial to the prescribed rate.

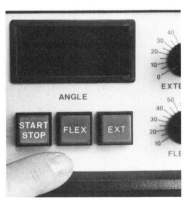

3 To operate the drive unit manually during setup, push the FLEX and EXT buttons.

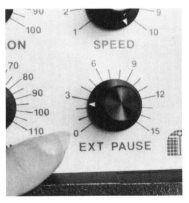

7 If ordered, use the EXT PAUSE button to direct the unit to pause a prescribed number of seconds when the leg's fully extended. *Note:* During the pause, the CPM device can activate a neuromuscular stimulator for the length of the pause. The stimulator attaches to the CPM device with an optional cable.

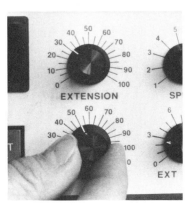

4 Adjust the FLEXION and EXTENSION dials to the ordered range of motion. *Note:* The equipment will shut down if you set EXTENSION higher than FLEXION or if you set the dials within 5 degrees of each other.

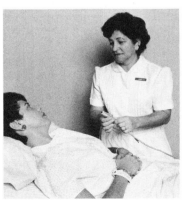

8 Show the patient how to use the patient control cord to stop and start the unit. Don't leave her alone until you've observed at least one full cycle.

Combating thrombosis with a sequential compression device

Edith Mayer, an 83-year-old widow, just had emergency surgery to repair a hip fracture. You know that deep vein thrombosis (DVT) occurs in half of all hip surgery patients and that this patient's advanced age puts her at additional risk. But by using a sequential compression device (SCD), you may help her avoid complications.

To prevent venous blood stagnation in Mrs. Mayer's legs, the doctor orders Kendall Company's T.E.D. Sequential Compression Device, illustrated below. Its components include a white and blue box called the controller; a pair of inflatable, three-chambered plastic sleeves (available in several sizes and lengths); and a Y-shaped tubing assembly that connects the sleeves to the controller.

Using compressed air, the controller systematically inflates and deflates each sleeve's three chambers, beginning at the ankle and moving up the leg. By doing so, it creates a wavelike milking action that nearly empties the veins and increases blood flow velocity in the femoral vein. The system operates on an automatically timed 71-second cycle: 11 seconds of compression followed by 60 seconds of decompression.

The controller acts as the system's brain and lungs. Its features include:
• a pressure adjustment knob for modifying pressures in sleeve compartments
• a digital display that shows pressure readings (in mm Hg) at every point in the inflation cycle
• a cycle monitor that continuously displays compression cycle status by representing the cycle's four phases—ankle, calf, thigh, and vent—on a lighted bar graph
• an audible alarm and automatic decompression, safety features that protect the patient if a pressure fault condition occurs.

Indications and contraindications

The doctor may order an SCD for any patient who, like Mrs. Mayer, faces a high risk of DVT because of age and prolonged immobility. He may also order an SCD to help prevent postoperative clotting complications in a patient who can't receive anticoagulant therapy (for example, because of a bleeding disorder).

Contraindications for SCD use include:
• a leg condition with which the sleeves would interfere (for example, dermatitis, a recent skin graft, or gangrene)
• recent leg vein ligation
• severe arteriosclerosis or other ischemic vascular disease
• massive leg edema or pulmonary edema from congestive heart failure
• severe leg deformity
• preexisting DVT (known or suspected).

Special considerations

Before using an SCD on the patient, make sure that all tubing connections are secure and that the tubing has no kinks or bends. Also check that the controller's back and bottom are unobstructed to allow free air flow and that its power cord is properly grounded.

If you're using a sleeve on only one of the patient's legs, connect the unused sleeve to the controller, according to the manufacturer's instructions, or the equipment won't work.

During therapy, check the patient's condition regularly. Remove the sleeves if she reports pain, numbness, or tingling in her legs. *Caution:* Don't operate the equipment near flammable anesthetic gases.

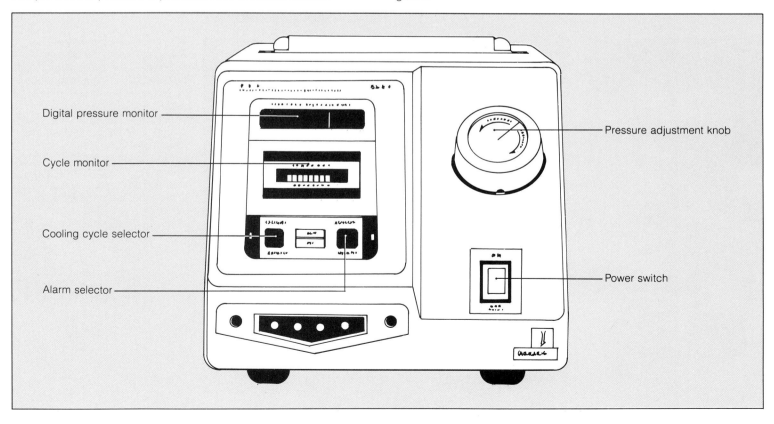

Digital pressure monitor — Pressure adjustment knob

Cycle monitor

Cooling cycle selector

Alarm selector — Power switch

Postoperative care

Setting up the T.E.D. Sequential Compression Device

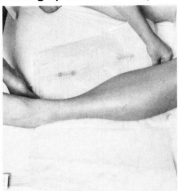

1 In this photostory, we'll feature thigh-length sleeves. Unfold the sleeve with the white side up and the narrower edge toward the foot. Then place the patient's leg on the sleeve, centering the blue line behind the knee.

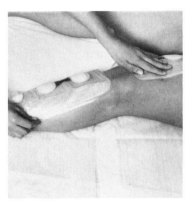

2 Starting with the side without Velcro or tubing, simultaneously wrap the ankle and thigh.

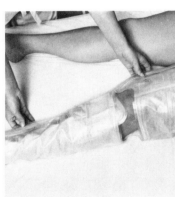

3 Secure the sleeve by firmly pressing the Velcro strip. Repeat the procedure to wrap the other leg. *Important:* Make sure the sleeves lie smoothly, without tucks or folds.

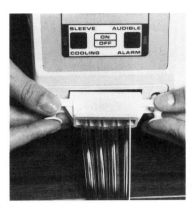

4 Attach the tubing assembly's larger plug to the controller.

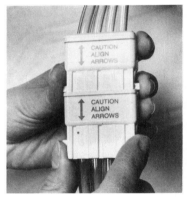

5 Then connect each sleeve's plug to the corresponding connector on the tubing assembly by squeezing in the latches on both sides, lining up the arrows, and pressing plug and connector together.
Turn on the controller's power switch. After performing self-diagnosis and lamp-check procedures, the controller begins operation with ankle chamber inflation.

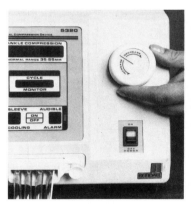

6 The digital display shows pressure in the sleeves throughout the cycle. After two or three cycles, pressure should be between 35 and 55 mm Hg. If necessary, adjust pressure by turning the knob above the power switch. One full clockwise turn lowers pressure about 5 to 7 mm Hg; one full counterclockwise turn raises pressure the same amount. Verify the adjusted pressure at the end of the next cycle.

Facts about the Mediscus Air Support Therapy System

Your patient returns to your unit after extensive surgery to repair traumatic injuries suffered in a motorcycle accident. Because he faces a long recovery period, he's at risk for such immobility hazards as pressure sores. How can you minimize problems?

The Mediscus Air Support Therapy System, a unique air-support bed, provides therapy for any immobilized patient. At the flick of a switch, filtered, warmed air flows through 21 low-friction, needle puncture-proof air sacs. The sacs evaporate perspiration and other moisture from the patient's immediate area; the warm air flowing through the sacs sweeps the moisture away. In this way, the system keeps the patient dry and helps prevent microorganisms from growing. Low air loss/constant air circulation protect the patient from dehydration.

The sacs also spread the patient's weight over a maximum support area, eliminating high pressure points and shear stresses, permitting good peripheral circulation, and preventing capillary closure. A patient who has pressure sores can rest comfortably without inhibiting the healing process.

Air enters the sacs on one side and leaves each sac via thru-put valves on the opposite side of the bed frame. When the patient moves and alters pressure points, the thru-put valve automatically compensates to maintain therapeutic pressure at all times.

The Mediscus system also:
• reduces the need to turn a patient every 2 hours, saving you time and minimizing the number of times you must disturb him
• relieves pain by providing support with less pressure than an ordinary mattress
• permits you to easily move a patient by sliding him across the low-friction air sacs
• deflates immediately to provide firm back support for cardiopulmonary resuscitation (see the photostory on page 103)
• deflates selectively to permit easy circumferential dressing changes, bedpan or incontinence pad placement, and wheelchair transfers. This feature eliminates the need to disturb the patient when performing a variety of procedures—for example, you can easily slide an X-ray plate behind the patient without lifting him.

The bed accommodates patients weighing up to 500 lb and measuring up to 6'9". Its accessories include attachments for all kinds of traction, proning sacs, cervical sacs, Hi-sacs (to prevent foot-drop), U-shaped sacs, and a bed scale. It can also provide traction for orthopedic patients.

When charting treatment, note that the patient's receiving air support therapy. Chart the time you placed the patient on the Mediscus Air Support Therapy System, the reason for therapy, and how the patient tolerated therapy. If he's being treated for a pressure sore, also chart wound size, location, drainage, odor, color, necrotic debris, and stage.

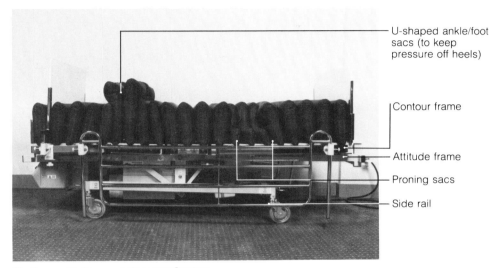

Mediscus Air Support Therapy System
The Mediscus bed's dual frame provides a variety of position options, including Trendelenburg's and reverse Trendelenburg's. When you elevate the head of the bed, the head section glides away from the seat section to allow full lung expansion, provide back support, stabilize the pelvic girdle, and eliminate shear forces. The patient can adjust the bed's position himself with the hand-held control (not shown).

Note the bars along the contour frame. They're color-coded to correspond to the five pressure gauges (shown below) that control pressure in each section of the five body areas: head, trunk, seat, thigh, and calf.

Control panel

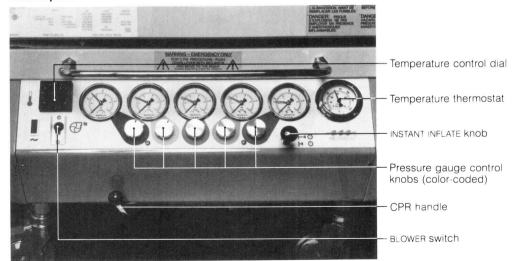

Postoperative care

How to use the Mediscus Air Support Therapy System

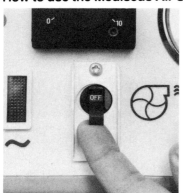

1 To start the system, insert the plug into an electrical outlet and flip the BLOWER switch on, as shown. A Mediscus service technician will adjust air sac pressures (as indicated by the green indicator needle on each pressure gauge) according to the patient's weight, height, and body distribution.

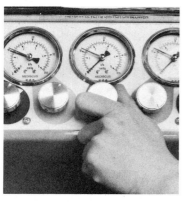

2 Now turn the color-coded knobs beneath the pressure gauges so that the black indicator needles align with the green indicator needles. This step ensures that all sections will deliver optimal therapeutic pressures.

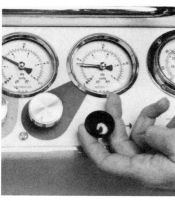

3 Before placing the patient on the bed, create maximum air sac pressures by lifting the INSTANT INFLATE knob, as shown. (When at maximum inflation, the bed is stretcher-height.)

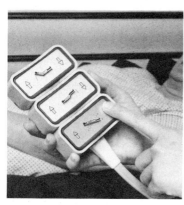

4 Slide and roll the patient onto the bed. Then use the hand-held control to put the bed in Trendelenburg's position.

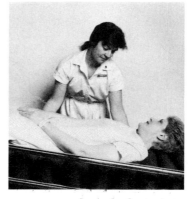

5 Put your hands under the patient's torso and slide her down toward the head of the bed, as shown here. (She slides easily across the air sacs.) Position her so that her iliac crest aligns with the red seat-section bar on the contour frame.

Using the hand-held control, reposition the bed as desired; then depress the INSTANT INFLATE knob to return the sacs to the preset therapeutic pressure.

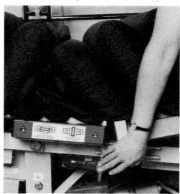

6 You can use this alternative method for transferring the patient to the bed: deflate the seat sacs by turning the red seat knob at the bed's side, as the nurse is doing here.

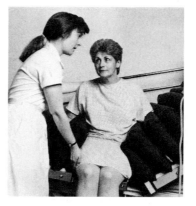

7 Then, sit the patient on the deflated seat sacs, as shown. Swing her legs onto the bed so that the deflated sacs cradle her pelvic girdle. Reinflate the seat sacs by turning the red lever.

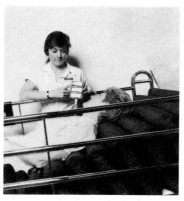

8 To sit the patient up, use the hand-held control to elevate the head of the bed (the contour frame inclines) and to lower the foot of the bed (the attitude frame declines).

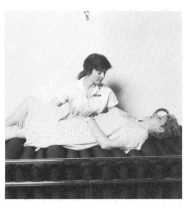

9 To turn the patient, use the hand-held control to position the bed horizontally. Lift the INSTANT INFLATE knob to achieve maximum pressure in all air sacs. Then turn the patient to a side-lying position.

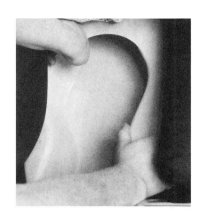

12 Use the same procedure if the patient needs to use a bedpan.

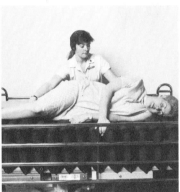

10 Cross one of the patient's legs over the other. To stabilize her, bend her upper leg slightly.
    Use a pillow to separate bony prominences, if necessary. Release the INSTANT INFLATE knob to return sac pressures to preset levels, and raise the side rails.

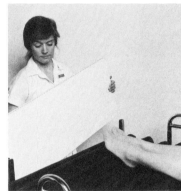

13 To transfer a patient who must maintain a prescribed degree of flexion, remove the footboard, as shown. Then remove the footboard's metal supports.

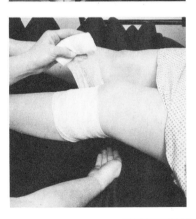

11 As this photo shows, you can deflate air sacs selectively to permit a circumferential dressing change. Release pressure in selected sacs by turning the pressure gauge knob that controls that section. (Remember, gauges are color-coded to correspond with the colored bars on the contour frame.)

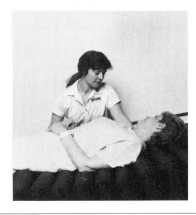

14 Place the bed in reverse Trendelenburg's position, and lift the INSTANT INFLATE knob to fully inflate the sacs. Then slide the patient down the bed, as the nurse is doing here.

How to clean Mediscus air sacs

The Mediscus bed has been designed for use without hospital linen (although you can use a cover sheet supplied by the manufacturer, if you wish). You can clean the air sacs easily while the patient remains in bed. Just move her to one side of the bed and sponge the air sacs with soap and water or a 1% disinfectant. Wipe off excess moisture and dry the sacs; then reposition the patient and repeat the procedure on the other side.

If a patient can't be moved, you can replace soiled sacs without disturbing her by twisting the air sac's two nylon connectors where they attach to the bed frame. You can do this when the patient's in bed, too.

To replace an air sac, push the air sac connectors back into the bed frame and listen for a clicking sound. Test the connection by gently pulling up on the sac.

Note: A Mediscus service technician regularly services the system and replaces all air sacs, vacuums debris, and cleans the air filter in accordance with Mediscus' infection control policy.

Postoperative care

Solving problems with the Mediscus Air Support Therapy System

Problem	Possible causes	Solutions
BED TEMP light comes on (some models).	• Temperature of air passing through air sacs has exceeded 106° F. • Room temperature too high; temperature in air sacs is approximately 10° F. warmer than room temperature.	• Turn off temperature control dial (0 position), which turns off heater. Light should go out in 30 minutes. If not, call Mediscus Service Center. • Decrease room temperature.
CHECK PRESSURES light comes on (some models).	• Air flow to air sacs is inadequate.	• Increase air sac pressures to recommended levels, as indicated by green arrows on pressure gauges; have air filter serviced.
Air sacs remain at maximum pressure.	• INSTANT INFLATE knob is engaged. • Pressure gauges set too high.	• Release INSTANT INFLATE knob. • Adjust pressure gauges to recommended levels, as indicated by green arrows on pressure gauges.
Blower won't start.	• No power at outlet • Thermal switch on motor inside has tripped.	• Check bed's plug. • Call Mediscus Service Center.
Bed won't tilt (Trendelenburg control inoperative).	• No power at outlet • Object blocking bed. • Hand control cord pinched.	• Check bed's plug. • Remove any object impeding bed movement. • Check hand control cord.
Head or foot contour won't move.	• Hand control cord pinched. • 4-amp breaker has tripped.	• Check hand control cord. • Call Mediscus Service Center.
Bed temperature won't increase.	• Temperature control set too low. • 7-amp heater circuit breaker has tripped.	• Increase temperature. • Call Mediscus Service Center.
Air sacs deflate, causing patient to sink to base of bed.	• Power failure	• During prolonged power failure, power pac will automatically engage.
Inadequate air pressure in sacs	• Voltage drop	• Power pac will automatically engage.

If your patient needs CPR

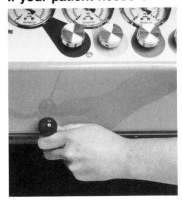

1 The Mediscus Air Support Therapy System responds quickly in a code situation. Slide the CPR valve (the lever with the red knob beneath the control panel) to your right, as the nurse is doing here.

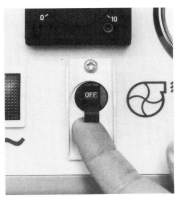

2 Then turn off the BLOWER switch and pull the bed's plug.

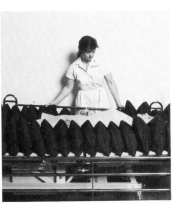

3 The air sacs deflate within 5 seconds, lowering the patient onto a firm back support. (If the bed wasn't horizontal initially, it levels automatically.) Lower the side rails.

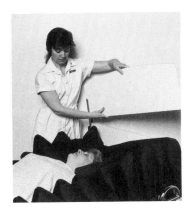

4 Then remove the headboard (to permit subsequent intubation) and begin CPR.

To restore air sac pressure after resuscitation, plug in the bed, return the CPR lever to its original position, and switch on the BLOWER.

Removing sutures with the Laschal Scissors

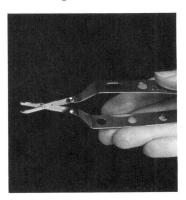

Have you ever wished for an extra hand while removing a patient's sutures? Now the Laschal Scissors, an inexpensive, easy-to-manipulate combination forceps/scissors instrument, allows you to grip, cut, and remove sutures in three precise movements, using one hand. With your other hand free, you can easily stabilize the incisional area or hold gauze for extracted sutures.

Here's how to use the Laschal Scissors:

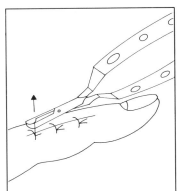

1 Use the scissors' forceps tip to elevate the suture tail and knot.

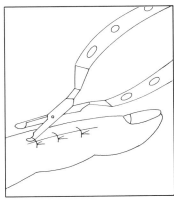

2 Next, gently engage the suture on the knot's right side, as shown. Cut the suture.

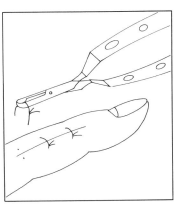

3 While the scissors remain closed, remove the suture and deposit it on the gauze in your free hand. Remove the remaining sutures in the same manner.

Note: To remove continuous or mattress sutures, use the Laschal Scissors as a conventional scissors to cut the sutures, then use the instrument to grasp and remove them.

Postoperative care

The ROHO Air Flotation System: An advance in pressure sore management

If your patient's confined to bed or a wheelchair, you constantly deal with the risk of pressure sores. By providing a cushion of flexible, low-pressure air cells between patient and bed or chairseat, a ROHO Air Flotation System product helps you manage this problem.

The ROHO heel pad featured here takes the pressure off an ischemic heel ulcer, improving blood flow to the area and promoting tissue healing. Designed for use without a cover, it's easily cleaned with antibacterial soap or low-sudsing detergent. It can also be sterilized in a gravitational displacement autoclave.

Besides the heel pad, ROHO, Inc. makes a variety of other air flotation products, including a mattress, cushion, and chair recliner. The company also offers a kit that allows you to customize a pad for your patient's needs. Here's how to apply the heel pad.

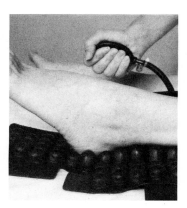

1 Lay the heel pad flat and inflate it fully, using the attached bulb pump. The cells should feel fairly stiff. Then, with the patient on his back, center his heel and Achilles tendon on the pad. *Note:* Don't let the heel rest on the pad's smaller rectangular portion.

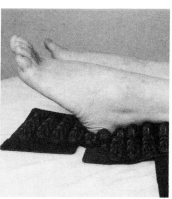

2 You'll note that with the cells fully inflated, the heel rides above the pad's shortest air cells. Now that you've positioned the heel, deflate the pad slightly until the heel depresses the shortest air cells to one half their full height. *Important:* Don't let the heel bottom out.

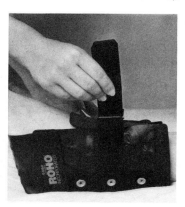

3 To wrap the foot, fold the heel flap up against the sole and attach its Velcro tabs to the ankle flaps. Then wrap the ankle flaps over the leg, pass the Velcro strap through the metal ring, adjust the strap for firmness, and fasten it against itself.

Preventing pressure sores: Your role

No matter how helpful, sophisticated equipment can't replace good nursing care. Frequently assess your patient's risk for ulcer formation, and share your findings with other team members. The following information discusses how to deal with each risk factor.

Pressure

When pressure on bony prominences exceeds 32 mm Hg, capillaries collapse and restrict blood flow.
To ease pressure:
• Reposition the patient at least every 2 hours.
• Provide skin care and massage.
• Use special beds, mattresses, or pads, such as the Mediscus bed and ROHO products featured in this section.

Friction

When skin moves against another surface, friction wears off the epidermal layer and may break compromised skin capillaries.
To reduce friction:
• Use sheepskin (in good condition).
• Apply elbow and heel protectors.
• Lower the head of the bed to less than 40 degrees, unless contraindicated.
• Apply skin sealants and skin barriers, such as transparent dressings; they protect the epidermis by acting as a second layer of skin.
• Use a lift sheet or lifting device to move the patient.
• Apply a light dusting of cornstarch under pendulous breasts and in other friction areas. (Don't use powder; it cakes and irritates.)

Shear

When a bony prominence slides along adjacent subcutaneous tissue, already-compromised capillaries constrict further.
To reduce shear:
• Use tape with an acrylate-based, nonallergenic adhesive. Avoid applying tape under tension, which creates shear and strips skin cells.
• Use skin sealants under tape.
• Use a lift sheet or lifting device to move the patient.
• Educate him about basic positioning principles.

Moisture

Excess moisture causes maceration and contributes to bacteria growth.
To prevent excess moisture:
• Keep the skin clean and dry. Use pH-balanced skin care products.
• Use incontinence devices, if indicated.

Other factors

Underlying disease and other factors relating to the patient's condition, including malnutrition and immobility, contribute to ulcer formation.
To manage conditions that favor ulcer formation:
• Ensure adequate nutritional and fluid intake.
• Work with the physical therapist to reduce immobility hazards.
• Combat skin dryness with emollient creams.
• Consult with the doctor about underlying disease.

Caring for the Critically Ill Patient

Cardiac care | Neurologic care | Organ donation
Respiratory care | Renal care

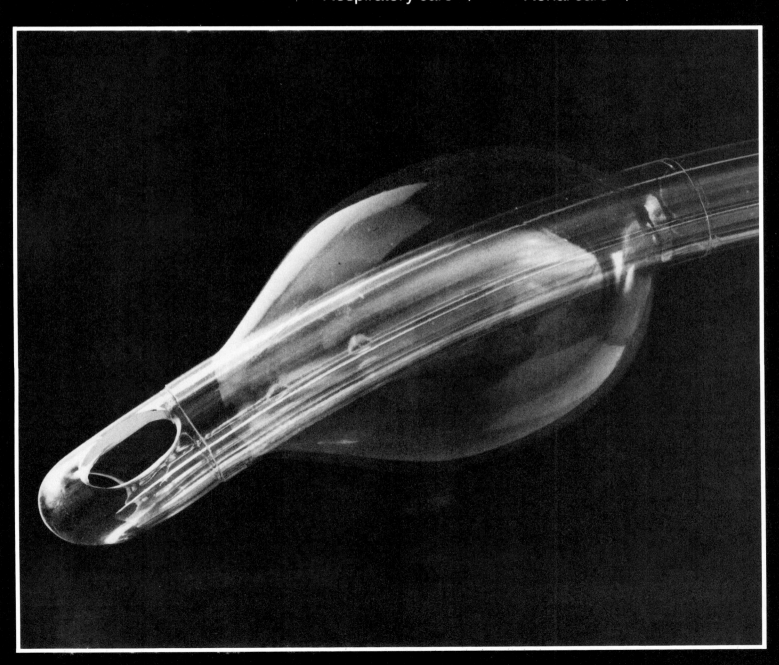

Cardiac care

Advances in diagnostics, drug therapy, and defibrillator equipment hold promise for many patients with life-threatening cardiac disorders. In the following pages, we'll discuss new cardiac drugs—and two new formulations for an old friend, nitroglycerin. We'll also show you two options for the ambulatory patient at risk for life-threatening ventricular dysrhythmias: an implantable defibrillator that delivers a shock immediately upon sensing ventricular tachycardia or fibrillation and an external advisory defibrillator that a patient's companion learns to use in an emergency. And finally, we'll acquaint you with the world's first rate-responsive, single-chamber pacemaker—a device that could improve the quality of life for many pacemaker patients.

Coronary artery disease: Diagnostic and treatment options

Two new techniques—apolipoprotein immunoassay and intravenous injection of an experimental drug—may make the future brighter for your patients with coronary artery disease.

The *apolipoprotein immunoassay* helps predict patients at risk for cardiovascular disease by measuring blood levels of two types of apolipoproteins: apo A-1 and apo B-100. Found within lipoprotein complexes, both carry triglycerides and cholesterol through the bloodstream. However, they differ in an important way: apo A-1 carries its load toward the liver for excretion, whereas apo B-100 deposits its cholesterol in body cells. In practical terms, this means that a high proportion of apo B-100 in the blood (compared to the apo A-1 level) increases the risk of arterial obstruction. If test results determine that your patient's at risk, the doctor can design a program of reduced cholesterol intake, anticholesterol medication, and lifestyle changes.

If coronary artery blood clots trigger acute myocardial infarction (MI), an experimental drug—*human tissue-type plasminogen activator (TPA)*—may save the patient's life. Injecting TPA during the early stages of an acute MI quickly dissolves coronary artery blood clots, thus preventing extensive and often fatal myocardial damage. According to recent research, TPA dissolves blood clots twice as fast as streptokinase does; it's also more specific for fibrin clots, less antigenic, and less likely to cause excessive bleeding or systemic anticlotting effects. And the procedure doesn't require cardiac catheterization—you can administer TPA by simple intravenous injection, thus saving precious time.

Cardiac drug update

Become familiar with the indications and recommended dosages for these new antiarrhythmic drugs *before* you administer them. For more information, consult package inserts or your latest drug reference.

Acebutolol (Sectral)

A cardioselective beta-adrenergic blocker that's less likely than many other beta blockers to produce adverse pulmonary reactions, bradycardia, or peripheral vascular complications
Indications
• Hypertension
• Ventricular premature beats
Dosage and administration
For mild to moderate hypertension, give 400 to 800 mg P.O. daily; for severe hypertension, give up to 1,200 mg daily in two divided doses; for ventricular premature beats, give 600 to 1,200 mg daily in two divided doses.

Nursing considerations
• Acebutolol is contraindicated for patients with persistently severe bradycardia, second- or third-degree heart block, overt cardiac failure, or cardiogenic shock.
• If possible, avoid using acebutolol in patients with bronchospastic conditions, such as asthma.
• Keep in mind that acebutolol may potentiate insulin-induced hypoglycemia and may mask some of its manifestations, such as tachycardia.
• Monitor the patient for adverse reactions, including fatigue, dizziness, headache, insomnia, nausea, dyspepsia, constipation, diarrhea, urinary frequency, and dyspnea.
• If ordered, administer acebutolol with a thiazide diuretic to manage hypertension.
• Emphasize to the patient the importance of complying with dosage instructions—severe complications can result if he stops taking the drug abruptly, especially if he has coronary artery disease or hyperthyroidism.

• Warn him against using over-the-counter cold preparations or nose drops without consulting his doctor or pharmacist—combining these with acebutolol can cause severe hypertension.

Amiodarone (Cordarone)

A Class III antiarrhythmic that prolongs the refractory period and repolarization; may be ordered to treat dysrhythmias resistant to other drug therapy
Indications
• Ventricular and supraventricular dysrhythmias, including recurrent supraventricular tachycardia (such as that which occurs with Wolff-Parkinson-White syndrome)
• Atrial fibrillation and flutter
• Ventricular tachycardia
Dosage and administration
Give a loading dose of 800 to 1,600 mg P.O. daily for 1 to 3 weeks, until initial therapeutic

response occurs. Maintenance dose: 200 to 600 mg P.O. daily. *Note:* I.V. administration is investigational.

Nursing considerations
• Use amiodarone cautiously if your patient has preexisting bradycardia or sinus node disease, conduction disturbances, severely depressed ventricular function, or marked cardiomegaly.
• Divide the oral loading dose into three equal doses, and give them with meals to minimize adverse gastrointestinal (GI) effects. Give the maintenance dose once daily or, if GI intolerance occurs, divided into two doses taken with meals.
• Monitor the patient for symptoms of pneumonitis (more likely if he takes more than 600 mg daily); also watch for headache, malaise, fatigue, bradycardia, hypotension, nausea, vomiting, photosensitivity, and muscle weakness. Such adverse effects become more likely with high doses, but they should resolve within 4 months of ending therapy.
• Teach the patient to instill methylcellulose ophthalmic solution during amiodarone therapy to minimize corneal microdeposits (which occur in most patients 1 to 4 months after therapy begins).
• Tell him to use a sunscreen to prevent photosensitivity.

Encainide (Enkaid)

A Class IC antiarrhythmic that blocks sodium channels in Purkinje fibers and the myocardium by slowing phase 0 depolarization, with little effect on either action potential duration or repolarization

Indications
• Life-threatening dysrhythmias, such as sustained ventricular tachycardia
• Symptomatic nonsustained ventricular tachycardia
• Frequent premature ventricular complexes

Dosage and administration
Give one 25-mg capsule three times daily, at approximately 8-hour intervals. If necessary after 3 to 5 days, increase the dosage to 35 mg three times daily. If this fails to cause a therapeutic response, increase the dosage again, after another 3 to 5 days, to 50 mg three times daily. *Caution:* Avoid rapid dose escalation.

Nursing considerations
• Give encainide cautiously to a patient with congestive heart failure (CHF) or congestive cardiomyopathy.
• Initiate cardiac monitoring before beginning drug therapy if your patient has sustained ventricular tachycardia, sinus node dysfunction, cardiomyopathy, or CHF, or if he'll receive 200 mg/day or more of encainide.

• Monitor the patient closely for ventricular tachycardia (or exacerbation of preexisting ventricular tachycardia), which develops most commonly in patients with histories of sustained ventricular tachycardia, cardiomyopathy, CHF, or sustained ventricular tachycardia with cardiomyopathy or CHF.
• If your patient has hypokalemia or hyperkalemia, don't give encainide until correcting the imbalance.

Flecainide (Tambocor)

A Class IC antiarrhythmic that suppresses premature ventricular contractions (PVCs) and manages some dysrhythmias that resist other drugs. However, its negative inotropic effect may cause or worsen CHF in some patients.

Indication
• Ventricular dysrhythmias

Dosage and administration
Give 100 mg P.O. every 12 hours initially. Increase the dosage to 150 mg every 12 hours for sustained ventricular tachycardia (to a maximum of 400 mg daily) or to 200 mg every 12 hours for symptomatic nonsustained ventricular tachycardia, couplets, or PVCs (to a maximum of 600 mg daily).

Nursing considerations
• Flecainide is contraindicated for patients with preexisting second- or third-degree atrioventricular (AV) block, right bundle-branch block associated with left hemiblock (unless the patient has a pacemaker), or cardiogenic shock.
• Plasma digoxin levels may increase if you give flecainide with digoxin; if you give flecainide with propranolol, levels of both increase.
• If your patient has hypokalemia or hyperkalemia, don't give flecainide until correcting the imbalance.
• Monitor the patient for adverse effects, which may include new or worsening dysrhythmias or CHF, dizziness, visual disturbances, dyspnea, headache, nausea, fatigue, palpitations, chest pain, asthenia, tremors, constipation, edema, and abdominal pain.
• Emphasize to the patient the importance of taking the drug as prescribed.

Mexiletine (Mexitil)

A Class IB antiarrhythmic that depresses phase 0 and shortens the action potential

Indication
• Refractory ventricular dysrhythmias, including ventricular tachycardia and PVCs

Dosage and administration
Give 200 to 400 mg P.O. (may be given with meals) initially, followed by 200 mg every 8 hours (dosage may be increased to 400 mg every 8 hours if necessary). The patient may

respond well to mexiletine every 12 hours; if so, give up to 450 mg every 12 hours, as ordered. Twice-a-day doses encourage compliance.

Nursing considerations
• Give mexiletine cautiously if your patient has CHF or sinus node disease.
• If the doctor orders a change from lidocaine to mexiletine, stop the lidocaine infusion when you given the first mexiletine dose. However, keep the infusion line open until the dysrhythmia appears to be under control.
• Monitor the patient for tremors (especially fine hand tremors), an early sign of mexiletine toxicity. If you note tremors, question him about dizziness, ataxia, and nystagmus, which develop as the drug's blood level increases. (Therapeutic blood levels range from 0.75 to 2 mcg/ml.)
• Monitor for other adverse effects, including diplopia, confusion, nervousness, headache, hypotension, bradycardia, nausea, vomiting, and skin rash.
• Monitor blood pressure, heart rate, and heart rhythm frequently. Notify the doctor of any significant change.

Tocainide (Tonocard)

A Class IB antiarrhythmic that depresses phase 0 and shortens the action potential

Indication
• Symptomatic ventricular dysrhythmias, including frequent PVCs and ventricular tachycardia

Dosage and administration
Give 400 mg P.O. every 8 hours initially. Then expect to give between 1,200 and 1,800 mg/day divided into three doses.

Nursing considerations
• Tocainide is contraindicated for patients hypersensitive to lidocaine or other amide-type local anesthetics and for those with second- or third-degree AV block in the absence of a ventricular pacemaker.
• Give tocainide cautiously if your patient has CHF or diminished cardiac reserve. As ordered, lower the dosage if he has hepatic or renal impairment.
• Give doses with food to minimize adverse GI effects.
• Monitor the patient for adverse effects, including light-headedness, tremors, hypotension, blurred vision, nausea, vomiting, epigastric pain, skin rash, and aplastic anemia. Tremors may indicate approach of the maximum dose. (Therapeutic blood levels range from 4 to 10 mcg/ml.) Adverse reactions are generally mild, transient, and reversible by reducing dosage.
• Protect the patient from falling if he becomes dizzy (a particular risk for elderly patients).

Cardiac care

Two new nitroglycerin formulations: A closer look

Angina sufferers now have two new alternatives to sublingual nitroglycerin tablets—nitroglycerin lingual aerosol (Nitrolingual Spray) and transmucosal controlled-release nitroglycerin tablets (Nitrogard). Before you give them, use the chart below to familiarize yourself with their indications and recommended dosages. Then make sure you provide your patient with appropriate guidelines for their use.

Nitroglycerin lingual aerosol (Nitrolingual Spray)	Transmucosal controlled-release nitroglycerin tablets (Nitrogard)
A metered-dose aerosol containing nitroglycerin in a propellant. The spray canister contains 200 metered 0.4-mg doses (the same dose as most sublingual tablets). Rapidly absorbed through the oral mucosa, the spray provides almost instant pain relief.	A controlled-release tablet that dissolves slowly when placed in a buccal pouch and is absorbed through the oral mucosa. It begins to release nitroglycerin on contact with the mucosa and continues to release the drug as it dissolves.
Indications	*Indications*
• To relieve acute angina attacks • To prevent exertion-induced angina	• To relieve acute angina attacks • To prevent exertion-induced angina
Dosage and administration	*Dosage and administration*
• To relieve acute angina, have the patient spray one 0.4-mg dose on or under his tongue, then close his mouth. (Warn him not to swallow immediately or to inhale the spray.) He can repeat the application in 3 to 5 minutes, but he shouldn't exceed three doses in 15 minutes.	• To relieve acute angina, have the patient place a tablet on the oral mucosa between his lip and gum above the upper incisors or between his cheek and gum, and tell him to allow it to dissolve slowly over 3 to 5 hours. (Warn him not to chew or swallow it.) The usual starting dose is 1 mg; the doctor may titrate this upward incrementally until an effective dose is reached or until side effects limit the dose. *Note:* If the recommended dose doesn't relieve an acute angina attack promptly, tell the patient to take sublingual nitroglycerin.
• To prevent angina, have the patient spray one dose on or under his tongue 5 to 10 minutes before he engages in strenuous activity.	• To prevent angina, have the patient insert one tablet (usually a 1-mg dose to start) every 5 hours during working hours or as ordered. The doctor may adjust the dosage upward to the next tablet strength if angina occurs while the tablet's in place. If angina occurs after the tablet dissolves, the doctor may increase dosage frequency—for example, to every 4 hours.
Nursing considerations	*Nursing considerations*
• The spray canister may be easier to handle than sublingual tablets during an acute angina attack, particularly for a sight-impaired, arthritic, or otherwise disabled patient. And the canister protects nitroglycerin from heat and light, preserving its potency for up to 3 years (some sublingual tablets remain potent for only 3 to 6 months). • Advise the patient to sit down when he applies the spray, to prevent postural hypotension. Also tell him to go to the hospital emergency department if his angina doesn't subside after treatment with the spray.	• Tell the patient to avoid using the tablets at bedtime because of the aspiration risk. • Tell him that he may talk, eat, and drink while the tablet's in place; warn him, however, that the tablet may dissolve faster if he drinks hot liquids or touches the tablet with his tongue. • Monitor the patient for adverse reactions, particularly headache and hypotension. He may have a headache during initial therapy, but a standard headache remedy or a dosage adjustment should relieve it, and it will probably disappear after the first week or two of therapy. Because the drug may cause postural hypotension, give it cautiously to a patient with volume depletion from diuretic therapy or with systolic blood pressure below 90 mm Hg.

VENTAK AICD: Preventive therapy for sudden cardiac death

By one estimate, 400,000 Americans will experience a sudden death episode this year; most (about 80%) won't survive. Many of the survivors will be candidates for the CPI VENTAK Automatic Implantable Cardioverter Defibrillator (AICD) shown at right.

The AICD generator rests in a subcutaneous or submuscular abdominal pocket. Relying on information from several leads—for example, a superior vena cava lead, a bipolar endocardial lead, and a ventricular patch lead—it identifies ventricular tachycardia (VT) and ventricular fibrillation (VF) in 5 to 20 seconds. Within 15 more seconds, it triggers a countershock. If necessary, it can generate up to four countershocks in sequence. (Depending on the VENTAK model, shocks measure 25 or 30 joules). After the fourth shock, the generator must recognize a regular rhythm for at least 35 seconds before it begins another four-shock cycle; however, most dysrhythmias convert with the first shock.

External equipment used with the AICD system includes the AIDCHECK interrogation device, the AIDCHECK probe, the CPI doughnut magnet, and the External Cardioverter Defibrillator (ECD), which is used during the implant procedure.

Indications

Patients most likely to benefit from AICD implantation include:
• survivors of sudden cardiac death not associated with acute myocardial infarction, whose inducible dysrhythmias can't be controlled by drug therapy
• patients who've experienced more than one cardiac arrest and whose dysrhythmias can't be induced
• sudden cardiac death survivors with prolonged Q-T syndrome
• patients with sustained hypotensive VT (for patient

comfort, the device is generally not recommended for patients who have frequent VT episodes that would trigger shocks when they're awake).

Among patients currently benefitting from a VENTAK AICD, nearly 75% have a primary diagnosis of arteriosclerotic heart disease. The next most common primary diagnosis is nonischemic cardiomyopathy. Other primary diagnoses include idiopathic ventricular dysrhythmias, valvular heart disease, and prolonged Q-T syndrome. In about one third of patients, congestive heart failure accompanies the primary diagnosis.

Nursing considerations
Before and after surgery, provide the same basic care you'd give to a patient receiving an implanted pacemaker. In addition:
• teach the patient and his family about the AICD—what it is and what it can do. Tell him what to expect if it delivers a countershock: he may feel like he's received a kick or blow to the chest. (Some patients feel palpitations, dizziness, or weakness before a shock; others have no symptoms.)
• provide emotional support by encouraging the patient to talk and ask questions—concern about receiving uncomfortable shocks may make him anxious. Emphasize that the device should deliver a shock only in response to a life-threatening dysrhythmia; afterward, he'll probably have a feeling of well-being.
• after surgery, closely monitor the patient's EKG. *Note:* Some standard computerized or nurse-initiated EKG monitoring systems fail to automatically record shocks, which they regard as artifact.
• if the patient experiences sustained VT or VF, follow the same emergency protocol you'd use for any patient. (External defibrillators won't damage VENTAK.) If external electrical countershock doesn't convert the dysrhythmia, changing the paddle configuration to anterior-posterior may succeed.
• inform him that strong magnetic fields may inactivate the generator. Tell him to present his AICD patient identification card or Medic Alert identification to airport security personnel, rather than submit to electronic frisking. (If he hears beeping tones from the VENTAK, he's in a magnetic field—he must leave the area at once.)
• discuss the possibility that another person (for example, the

patient's wife) may feel a shock if she's touching the patient when the AICD discharges. However, the shock won't harm her.
 Nursing tip: If you're caring for a patient who's receiving frequent shocks, protect yourself by wearing rubber gloves.
• if the patient should feel dizzy, tell him to lie down and summon help immediately, without waiting for the AICD to discharge. If he loses consciousness, his family or companions should call for help, unlock the doors, and begin cardiopulmonary resuscitation.
• urge him to keep all follow-up appointments. The equipment needs checking every other month for the first year after implantation and once a month thereafter.
• encourage him to notify the doctor any time he receives a shock. He should also keep a diary of the date, time, and symptoms associated with each episode and share it with the doctor.

VENTAK AICD
Shown here with the VENTAK generator: small and large patch leads, a superior vena cava lead (the thicker metal lead), and a bipolar endocardial lead.

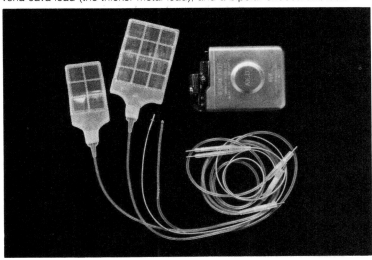

Magnet testing: Follow-up care for AICD patients
A patient who has a VENTAK AICD undergoes regular noninvasive magnet tests to determine battery status and the number of shocks the device has delivered. If you're performing the test, you'll use a CPI doughnut magnet (which also activates or inactivates the device) and an AID-CHECK interrogator with probe.

To use the AIDCHECK system, follow these steps:
• Palpate to locate the implanted AICD generator.
• Apply the AIDCHECK probe over the generator's upper left corner (as viewed from the front) and the magnet over the generator's upper right corner (see photo). You may tape the probe in place if you wish.
• Hold the magnet in place for at least 2 seconds (but no longer than 25 seconds).
• Leaving the probe in place, remove the magnet and listen for AIDCHECK to emit tones.
• Read and record the charge time and patient pulse count displayed by the AIDCHECK interrogator.

• Deactivate/reactivate VENTAK (see the following information); then wait 10 to 30 minutes and perform another magnet test.

How to deactivate/reactivate VENTAK
After any magnet maneuver, deactivate/reactivate VENTAK with this procedure:
• Place the magnet over the generator's upper right corner for 30 seconds, then remove it. (Make sure the probe remains in place.) You'll hear pulsed tones synchronous with R waves for 30 seconds, then a constant tone that indicates deactivation.
• Wait 10 seconds; then, with the probe in place, reactivate VENTAK by replacing the magnet over the generator's upper right corner for 30 seconds. You'll hear a constant tone for 30 seconds, followed by a few random tones and then R-wave synchronous tones (indicating an active implanted generator).
• If you accidentally perform a magnet test during the deactivate/reactivate procedure, repeat the procedure.

Note: Avoid unnecessary magnet maneuvers. Follow the manufacturer's recommendations.

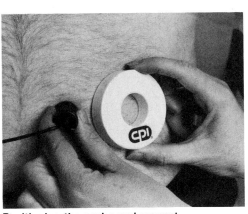

Positioning the probe and magnet

Cardiac care

LIFEPAK 100 Automatic Advisory Defibrillator: An innovation in home care

Now, a patient at risk for sudden cardiac death has an alternative to the automatic implantable cardioverter defibrillator featured on the preceding pages. The doctor may prescribe Physio-Control Corporation's lightweight LIFEPAK 100, an automatic advisory defibrillator that the patient's spouse or companion can use (along with cardiopulmonary resuscitation) if the patient suffers cardiac arrest. Equipped with a soft carrying case and shoulder strap, it can accompany the patient everywhere.

After the doctor prescribes the device, the patient's spouse or companion completes a training program. Then, if the patient suffers cardiac arrest, she opens the case and places the device's electrodes on the patient's chest (see the following photostory for details on the procedure). LIFEPAK 100 analyzes the patient's cardiac rhythm and determines whether he needs defibrillation. Its display screen then instructs the rescuer either to begin CPR or to administer a shock.

Designed for use by lay people, LIFEPAK 100 is intended to augment (not replace) conventional emergency response systems. The rescuer needs no EKG interpretive skills to use it.

Most people complete training in a few hours. The manufacturer recommends periodic refresher courses for long-term users and provides a review booklet and user guide for review between sessions.

Features
LIFEPAK 100 will deliver a shock only if these four conditions occur in sequence:
• the rescuer indicates that the patient isn't conscious
• the device detects no patient movement during EKG analysis
• the device detects a shockable rhythm during EKG analysis
• the rescuer presses the SHOCK button when advised to do so.

During use, LIFEPAK 100 keeps a record of each event, including elapsed time, EKG strips analyzed during the event, and the number of shocks delivered. After use, it must be returned to the manufacturer, who replaces the battery and electrodes, generates an episode report (based on the device's record of the event), and issues a formal report to the prescribing doctor.

Special considerations
• Don't open the device except to use it. (A battery test card permits periodic battery checks without opening the device.)
• Use the device only on the patient for whom it's been prescribed.
• Don't use it on a patient with a cardiac pacemaker, on a child, or on anyone weighing less than 80 lb (36 kg).
• Don't expose it to temperature extremes or immerse it in water. (However, it can be used safely in the rain, if necessary.)
• Return it for servicing after opening it for any reason (or before its expiration date, if it hasn't been opened).

Using a LIFEPAK 100 external defibrillator

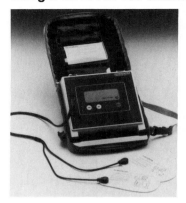

1 This portable defibrillator, designed for use with CPR, has a message display screen with YES and NO response buttons and a shock control. The equipment also includes self-adhesive defibrillation electrodes, an electrode cable, and scissors (to cut clothing, if necessary). LIFEPAK 100 should be used only by those trained to use it. *Important:* LIFEPAK 100 is factory-sealed. Don't open it unless the patient for whom it's prescribed collapses.

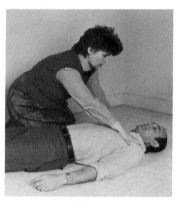

2 If the patient collapses, the rescuer must first make sure he's in cardiac arrest. Following standard CPR procedure, she establishes unresponsiveness by shaking and shouting; opening the airway; looking, listening, and feeling for breathing; giving ventilations; and checking for pulse.

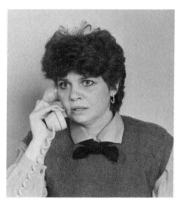

3 Having established unresponsiveness, she next calls the local emergency number and summons help.

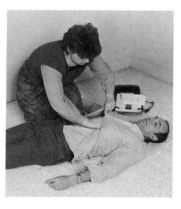

4 With the patient on his back on a firm surface, she places the equipment near his side and opens the case. She then removes all clothing from his chest, using the scissors in the case if necessary.

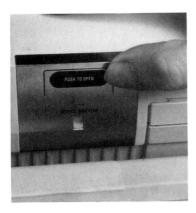

5 After wiping the patient's skin dry, she opens the defibrillator unit by pressing the upper part of the tab labeled PUSH TO OPEN and removing the lid.

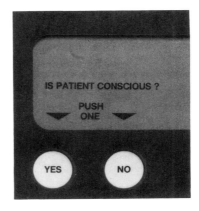

9 Responding to the screen's query, *IS PATIENT CONSCIOUS?*, she again shakes the patient and shouts, "Are you OK?" When he doesn't respond, she presses the NO button.

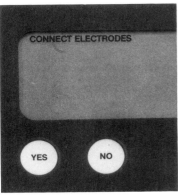

6 The message screen says *CONNECT ELECTRODES.*

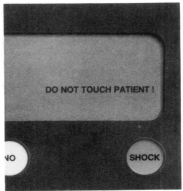

10 As the device analyzes the patient's cardiac rhythm, the screen instructs the rescuer to avoid touching the patient. If the device senses patient movement, it suspends EKG analysis.

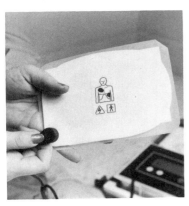

7 The rescuer opens the electrode package contained in the unit, snaps the cables to the electrodes, and removes the electrode backing.

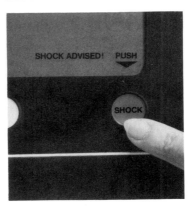

11 If the device advises defibrillation, the screen says *SHOCK ADVISED.* The rescuer presses the SHOCK button and moves clear of the patient. The device charges and delivers a shock in about 12 seconds while emitting a warning tone.

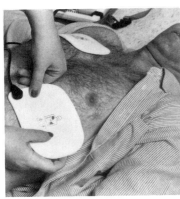

8 Pressing firmly around the electrode edges, she applies the electrodes, as shown.

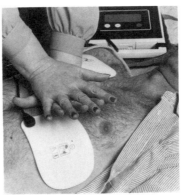

12 After the device delivers a shock, the screen instructs the rescuer to deliver 2 breaths and 15 chest compressions. The rescuer can begin CPR immediately, as instructed, without first checking for a pulse. The screen asks her to press the YES button when she completes CPR (see the first photo on the following page).

Cardiac care

Using a LIFEPAK 100 external defibrillator continued

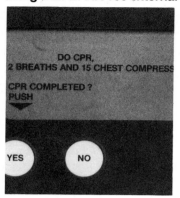

13 When the rescuer presses YES in response to the query shown here, the cycle begins again with the screen asking, *IS PATIENT CONSCIOUS?* If she presses NO, the device repeats analysis and advises her whether to give another shock. If it doesn't advise a shock, it provides instructions—for example, *DO CPR.* (The device won't respond if she presses the SHOCK button against its recommendation.)

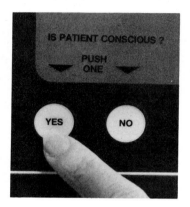

14 If the patient regains consciousness, the rescuer presses the YES button in response to the query. The query will remain on the screen. She shouldn't remove the electrodes until help arrives.

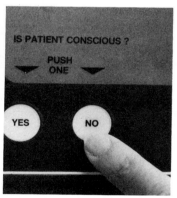

15 If the patient later loses consciousness, the rescuer presses the NO button and the device again analyzes his cardiac rhythm.

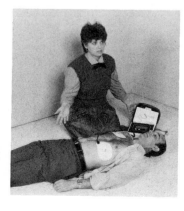

16 When emergency personnel arrive, the rescuer explains that the equipment is an automatic advisory defibrillator and tells them how many shocks have been delivered (if any). The manufacturer recommends informing local emergency organizations that the patient has LIFEPAK equipment before an emergency occurs.

The Activitrax pacemaker: Keeping pace with an active patient

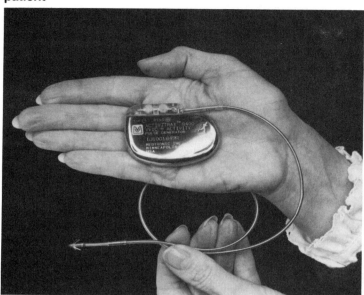

Like most patients with conventional single-chamber pacemakers, Roy Dolenz frequently found himself breathless and tired after even moderate bursts of activity. His pacemaker's fixed rate—70 beats/minute—wouldn't even permit him to take the long, brisk walks he used to enjoy.

Not long ago, however, Mr. Dolenz received a new pacemaker designed to respond to increases in physical activity: Activitrax, the world's first rate-responsive, single-chamber pacemaker. Now he can be as active as he wishes without fear of becoming breathless or dizzy. He says he feels healthier than he has in years.

A unique design
How does Activitrax work? A pressure-sensing quartz crystal bonded to the inside of the pacemaker's titanium shell detects even subtle pressure waves from physical activity. It then produces an electrical current that signals the pacemaker to increase heart rate appropriately. Activitrax can maintain heart rate within a broad range—from 60 to 150 beats/minute.

The doctor implants Activitrax in the same way he'd implant any single-chamber pacemaker. If he's replacing a patient's conventional VVI pacemaker, he can simply connect Activitrax to the previously implanted lead.

Almost any patient who needs a single-chamber pacemaker can benefit from Activitrax. Patients who won't benefit include:
• chronically bedridden patients
• patients with functional sinus nodes, who are better served by dual-chamber pacing.

Programming parameters
The doctor programs amplitude, pulse width, and sensitivity in the same way he'd program any VVI pacemaker, using standard programming equipment supplied by the manufacturer (Medtronic, Inc.). In addition, he must program four variables specific to rate-responsive pacing. You should be aware of these variables if you're caring for a patient with an Activitrax pacemaker.
• *Basic rate,* the minimum heart rate (60, 70, or 80 beats/minute)
• *Maximum activity rate,* the highest heart rate Activitrax can stimulate (100, 125, or 150 beats/minute)

• *Activity threshold,* the activity level that the patient must exceed before Activitrax increases heart rate (low, medium, and high). The threshold settings let Activitrax respond to certain activities (such as walking) that exceed the threshold, while ignoring others.
• *Rate response.* The doctor can program Activitrax to any one of 10 response settings to determine the paced rate that will occur at a given activity level.

Although the doctor can choose among 30 combinations of rate response and activity threshold settings, most patients do best on a basic combination suggested by the manufacturer. The variety of choice allows the doctor to fine-tune the system to suit an unusually active (or inactive) patient.

Special considerations
Because Activitrax responds to vibration, its circuitry contains special filters that screen out environmental influences from electrical appliances and even gardening equipment. It's designed to ignore vibrations from a bumpy car ride and continue functioning within normal limits.

The doctor may screen out unusually strong work-related vibrations (for example, from heavy machinery) by programming Activitrax at the high activity setting. But this depends on the patient—if he works hard, he needs a more responsive heart rate.

Tell your patient to report any problems to the doctor. His Activitrax may need reprogramming if he:
• experiences fatigue or shortness of breath during normal activities.
• experiences palpitations.
• changes his life-style or increases his activity level (many patients gradually become more active after Activitrax implantation, requiring adjustment in rate response and rate limit).
• experiences angina at high heart rates.
• undergoes a change in his medical condition.

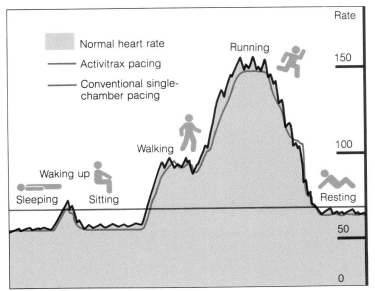

Unlike a conventional single-chamber pacemaker, the Activitrax pacemaker responds to increased physical activity by raising heart rate. As this graph shows, Activitrax pacing closely approximates a normal heart's response to activity.

ICHD codes
A pacemaker coding system devised by the Intersociety Commission for Heart Disease (ICHD) clearly identifies pacemaker capabilities. The code's five letters have the following significance:
• The first letter signifies the heart chamber being paced: V (ventricle), A (atrium), or D (dual, or both chambers).
• The second letter identifies the heart chamber the pacemaker senses: A, V, D, or O (none or not applicable).
• The third letter indicates how the pacemaker generator responds to the sensed event: T (triggered), I (inhibited), D (both triggered and inhibited), O (not applicable), or R (reverse).
• The fourth letter shows available programmable functions.
• The fifth letter indicates how the pacemaker reacts to tachydysrhythmia.

Keep in mind, though, that most pacemaker codes have only three letters, which refer to the first three variables.

Guide to pacemaker codes

Letter position				
1 Chamber paced	**2** Chamber sensed	**3** Mode of response	**4** Programmable functions	**5** Tachydysrhythmia function

Letters used				
V: Ventricle	V: Ventricle	T: Triggered	P: Programmable (rate and/or output only)	B: Bursts
A: Atrium	A: Atrium	I: Inhibited	M: Multiprogrammable	N: Normal rate competition
D: Dual	D: Dual	D: Dual O: None	C: Communicating	S: Scanning
	O: None	R: Reverse	O: None	E: External

Respiratory care

How much do you know about pulse oximetry? This noninvasive monitoring system provides continuous information about arterial oxygen saturation without subjecting the patient to a painful arterial stick.

That's just one of the recent advances in respiratory care that we cover here. Other new equipment featured in this section includes:
• PressureEasy cuff-pressure controller for maintaining correct endotracheal tube cuff pressures
• CyberSet speech system, which allows intubated patients to speak
• Trach Care closed tracheal suction system
• SleepEasy II nasal CPAP system for patients suffering from sleep apnea
• Bronchitrac "L" for easy suctioning of the left main stem bronchus.

We also acquaint you with two new ventilators that your patients may be using in the near future.

Pulse oximetry: Painless hypoxemia monitoring

Until recently, monitoring your patient's arterial oxygen status meant performing frequent arterial sticks or using a transcutaneous oxygen (tcPO$_2$) monitor. Now, pulse oximetry offers a reliable alternative to painful, time-consuming arterial sticks and the difficult-to-use tcPO$_2$ monitor.

Using light to measure arterial oxygen saturation (SaO$_2$), the pulse oximeter tracks your patient's SaO$_2$ level noninvasively and continuously—and monitors pulse rate and amplitude, too. Here's how the oximeter works:

Light-emitting diodes in a transducer (sensor) you attach to the patient's body send red and infrared light beams through tissue (see the illustration on page 117). A photodetector records the relative amount of each color absorbed by arterial blood and transmits the data to a monitor, which displays the information with each heartbeat. If the SaO$_2$ level or pulse rate exceeds or drops below user preset limits, visual and audible alarms go off.

The oximeter eliminates the delay associated with laboratory analysis of blood specimens; because it alerts you to abnormalities instantly, you can take immediate steps to correct them. Unlike the tcPO$_2$ monitor, it doesn't require warm-up time, calibration, or frequent location changes. And it can't burn the patient because it doesn't use heat.

To use the pulse oximeter shown below—Nellcor Inc.'s Nellcor N-100—you'll apply an oxygen transducer to your patient. Depending on his age, size, and clinical condition, you'll use one of these six oxygen transducers:
• neonatal foot transducer
• infant toe transducer
• pediatric finger transducer
• adult finger transducer for patients engaging in limited activity
• adult nasal transducer for inactive patients (typically used during surgery)
• reusable adult finger transducer for patients needing only short-term, nonsterile monitoring.

Whenever possible, attach the adult finger transducer to the patient's index finger and keep the finger at heart level. Don't attach any transducer to an extremity that has a blood pressure cuff or an arterial catheter in place; occluded blood flow will hinder transducer performance. If the transducer's exposed to bright sunlight or other strong light, cover it completely with a towel or blanket. After you've attached the transducer, check it frequently to make sure it hasn't been damaged or displaced, and examine the skin site for abrasion and circulatory impairment.

To learn how to apply an adult finger transducer, read the following photostory.

Nellcor N-100 pulse oximeter

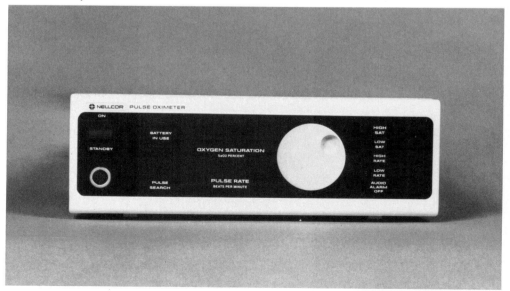

Applying an Oxisensor adult finger transducer

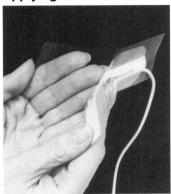

1 Obtain an Oxisensor adult digit oxygen transducer (model D-25) and remove its backing.

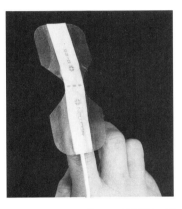

2 Place the transducer, adhesive side up, over the patient's finger. Position the dashed center line directly above the fingertip, as shown in this photo.

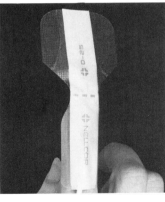

3 Press the transducer onto the patient's finger, and wrap the adhesive flaps on either side of the Nellcor label around the finger.

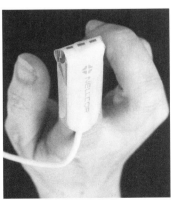

4 Now fold the transducer's other end under the patient's finger so that the two blue alignment marks directly oppose each other across his finger. Then wrap the adhesive flaps on the second side of the transducer around his finger. (To learn how to connect the transducer to the Nellcor N-100 pulse oximeter, read the following photostory.)

Setting up the Nellcor N-100 pulse oximeter

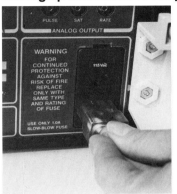

1 Plug the oximeter's power cord into the monitor, as shown, then into a grounded 100v or 120v AC outlet marked *Hospital only* or *Hospital grade.* (During an external power loss or a disconnection, an internal battery will power the oximeter automatically for up to 1 hour. If this happens, the BATTERY IN USE signal will light steadily, then flash when only a few minutes of battery operation remain.)

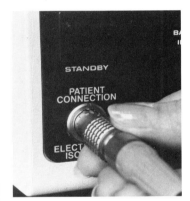

2 Connect the patient module to the oximeter by lining up the red dots on the cable connector with those in the socket, as shown here. Push the connector straight in until it locks (*don't* twist the connector while attaching or removing it).

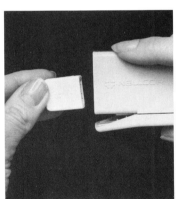

3 Plug the connector from the transducer (which you previously applied to the patient's finger, as described in the preceding photostory) into the oximeter's patient module.

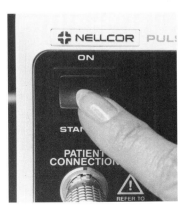

4 Turn the ON/STANDBY switch to the ON position. If the device is working properly, you'll hear a beep and see the displays light momentarily and the pulse search light flash. The SaO_2 and pulse rate displays show stationary zeros.

Respiratory care

Setting up the Nellcor N-100 pulse oximeter continued

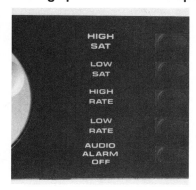

5 Check the alarm limits by pressing the row of buttons on the right front panel, shown here. (For more information on alarm limits, see page 117.)

The pulse amplitude indicator (a vertical light bar) reflects the strength of pulse perfusion. For an adult, the light normally rises at least halfway up the bar when the machine's first turned on.

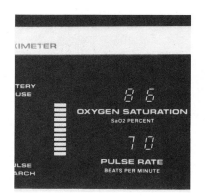

6 After four to six heartbeats, the SaO_2 and pulse rate displays will begin to show information with each beat and the pulse amplitude indicator begins to track the pulse. You'll also hear a beep, rising in pitch as SaO_2 increases and falling as SaO_2 decreases, with each beat.

How to adjust the pulse oximeter's alarm limits

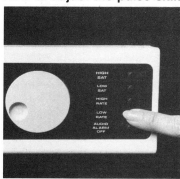

1 To adjust an alarm limit, depress the corresponding button; the current alarm limit appears in the display for 3 seconds. In this photo, the nurse has pressed the LOW RATE button to display the current low pulse rate setting, which in this case is *55*.

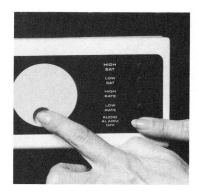

4 To silence the audio alarm for more or less than 60 seconds, hold the AUDIO ALARM OFF button while turning the control wheel to the desired setting (from 30 to 120 seconds, indicated in the display window). Then release the button.

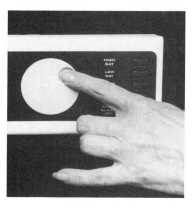

2 Suppose you want to lower the setting to 50. After you press the LOW RATE button, rotate the control wheel counterclockwise. Stop rotating the wheel when *50* appears in the pulse rate window. (To raise the limit, turn the wheel clockwise.) The new limit remains in the window for 3 seconds; then the display again shows current pulse and SaO_2 values. (When you turn off the monitor, alarm limits revert to preset levels.)

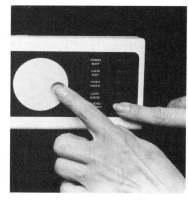

5 To turn the audio alarm off completely, depress the AUDIO ALARM OFF button and turn the control knob to the right beyond the 120-second interval. The word *OFF* appears on the SaO_2 display until you release the button, and the AUDIO ALARM OFF light begins flashing. Then you can turn the audio alarm on or off by depressing the AUDIO ALARM OFF button. (Never turn off the audio alarm if doing so would compromise patient safety.)

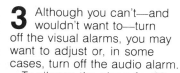

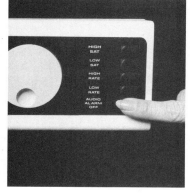

3 Although you can't—and wouldn't want to—turn off the visual alarms, you may want to adjust or, in some cases, turn off the audio alarm.

To silence the alarm for 60 seconds, press the AUDIO ALARM OFF button (located below the four alarm limit buttons), as shown. The red indicator light will come on to show that the audio alarm has been turned off. After 60 seconds, the alarm will automatically go back on and the indicator light will go off.

Learning about the pulse oximeter's alarm limits

The Nellcor N-100 oximeter has two sets of pre-set alarm limits, as follows.
For an adult:
- high oxygen saturation (SaO_2): 100%
- low SaO_2: 85%
- high pulse rate: 140 beats/minute
- low pulse rate: 55 beats/minute.
For a neonate:
- high SaO_2: 95%
- low SaO_2: 80%
- high pulse rate: 200 beats/minute
- low pulse rate: 100 beats/minute.

To check whether the N-100 is set for an adult or a neonate, press the HIGH SAT button after turning on the N-100. If the display shows *100*, the instrument is set for an adult. If it shows *95*, it's set for a neonate.

When the SaO_2 level or pulse rate exceeds or drops below the alarm limits, the corresponding indicator light and SaO_2 display on the front panel flash and the audio alarm sounds steadily (unless you've turned it off). *Note:* Loss of pulse signal or transducer connection also causes the audio alarm to sound. In this case, however, the SaO_2 and pulse rate displays go blank and the PULSE SEARCH indicator flashes.

The photostory on page 116 shows you how to adjust preset alarm limits.

How pulse oximetry works
As shown below, two diodes send red (visible) and infrared light beams through tissue. A photodetector determines the relative amount of color absorbed by arterial blood; this data indicates arterial hemoglobin saturation.

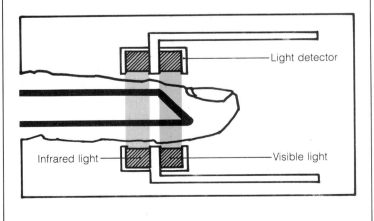

Light detector

Infrared light

Visible light

Suctioning with the Bronchitrac "L"

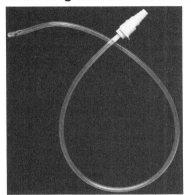

1 Suctioning a patient's left main stem bronchus sometimes poses a problem—the left bronchus is narrower than the right and veers away more sharply from the trachea. The Bronchitrac "L" suction catheter has a special design that makes suctioning easier. Because it enters the left bronchus automatically, it eliminates the need for patient repositioning and minimizes the risk of trauma to the patient.

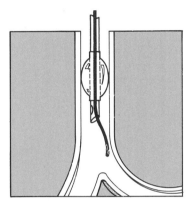

2 Remove the Bronchitrac from the package and lubricate its distal end with sterile water. Then insert the distal end into the patient's endotracheal (ET) tube. As you advance it, the catheter automatically points toward the left bronchus (see illustration).

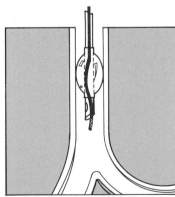

3 If you have trouble advancing it, the tip may have caught on the ET tube's side port. Withdraw the Bronchitrac slightly and rotate the proximal end one-eighth to one-quarter turn. Then carefully readvance it.

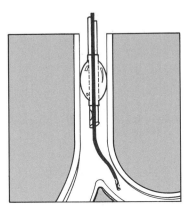

4 Continue advancing the Bronchitrac until it enters the left bronchus. If necessary, rotate the catheter's proximal end slightly. *Important:* If you encounter unexplained resistance at any point during catheter insertion, remove the Bronchitrac. *Never* force it.

With the catheter tip in the left bronchus, suction normally, keeping the proximal slide cover closed or slightly open.

Respiratory care

How to use the PressureEasy automatic cuff-pressure controller

If you're a critical care nurse, you're familiar with the complications that can occur with endotracheal (ET) tube use. Cuff overinflation can damage the patient's trachea; underinflation may cause vomitus aspiration. Ineffective sealing during peak flow can lead to another common problem—underventilation.

A cuff-pressure controller, such as the PressureEasy automatic cuff-pressure controller shown on this page, helps prevent such problems. Consider its advantages:
* *automatically maintains cuff pressure below 27 cmH₂O during expiration, protecting the tracheal wall, cilia, and mucosa*
* *keeps cuff pressure sufficiently above airway pressure (at approximately 25 cmH₂O), providing a safe, effective seal while inhibiting aspiration*
* *allows rapid cuff inflation, ensuring patient safety during initial and extended intubation*
* *provides continuous visual monitoring, eliminating the need for risky, repetitive cuff-pressure checks*
* *adapts to cuff volume changes while maintaining constant pressure, avoiding pressure changes caused by tracheal expansion*
* *regulates cuff pressure continuously, reducing the need for spot checks*
* *eliminates the need for fragile gauges and sensitive electronic devices, thus saving money.*

Learn how to assemble and use the PressureEasy automatic cuff-pressure controller by reading this photostory.

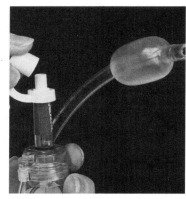

3 As you inject and release air, check for proper air flow through the inflation valve by watching the green stripe. It should move forward during injection, then partially retreat as air moves into the cuff. Once the stripe stabilizes in the safe range window, squeeze the pilot balloon; the stripe should move as air from the balloon and reservoir mix. Replace the valve cap. (Except during inflation and deflation, keep the valve cap in place.)

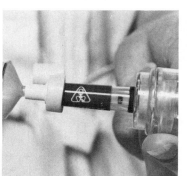

4 After your patient has been intubated and you've confirmed proper tube placement, inflate the PressureEasy valve by repeating Steps 2 and 3. Adjust pressure to the safe range.

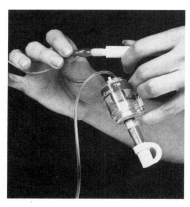

1 Locate the white cylindrical sleeve at the end of the short tube leading from the valve assembly. Press the sleeve securely over the inflation valve at the end of the patient's cuffed endotracheal tube; this activates the valve mechanism and prevents leakage.

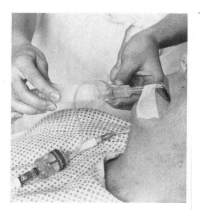

5 If your patient's receiving positive-pressure ventilation, attach PressureEasy's pressure feedback line to prevent blow-by leakage past the cuff. Connect the feedback adapter to the ET tube's 15-mm adapter. Press the adapter securely in place to adjust intracuff pressure during inspiration. Then attach the ventilator tubing, as shown. *Important:* Don't reuse PressureEasy with another patient after using it with the feedback line attached.

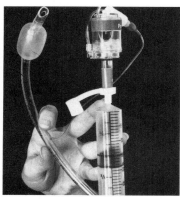

2 Now perform a test inflation. First, remove the cap from the PressureEasy valve. Using a 10-ml or larger syringe, inject enough air into the valve so that the green stripe on the end of the reservoir stem appears between the black label and the valve body in the safe range window. Check the valve and tube for leakage. Then release all air from the valve and cuff until you feel a vacuum within the syringe.

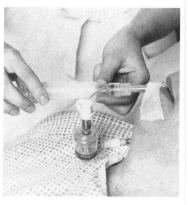

6 To prevent fluid accumulation in the valve when using the feedback line, position the feedback adapter so that the line faces upward, and pass the line through the valve cap's loop so that the valve hangs upside down, as shown. This allows fluid to pump back out of the valve automatically.

Trach Care closed suction system: A solution to common suctioning problems

If you've ever used a standard open suction system, you know that interrupting ventilation to perform suctioning can cause problems—for example, hypoxemia, dysrhythmias, hypotension, and increased intracranial pressure. Open suction also puts you at risk for infection from the patient's secretions.

By eliminating the need to disconnect the patient from the ventilator during suctioning, a closed suction system helps prevent such complications. Ballard Medical Products' Trach Care contains a specially designed T-piece that comes between the ventilator and the patient's tracheal or endotracheal tube to permit continuous ventilation. Because it becomes part of the ventilator circuit, the Trach Care system requires one setup procedure and change after 24 hours of use. Although the Trach Care catheter is repeatedly reintroduced into the patient's airway, studies show no significant difference in contamination rate when compared to an open system.

The Trach Care system offers these variations:
• adult, pediatric, and neonatal, French sizes 18, 16, 14, 12, 10, 8, and 6
• directional tip, French size 14 only.

To learn how to set up the Trach Care system, read the following photostory.

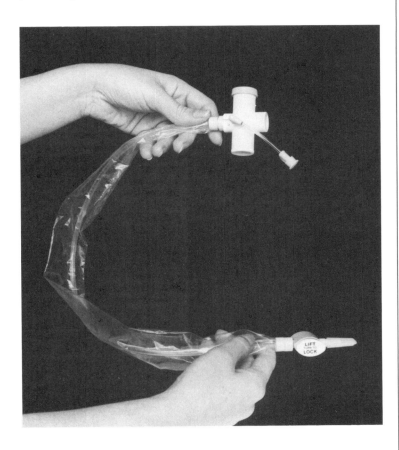

Using Trach Care closed suction system

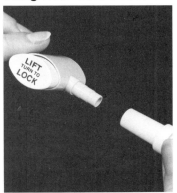

1 Remove the Trach Care system from the package and attach its thumb suction control valve to the wall suction tubing.

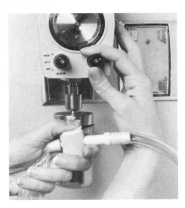

2 Depress the thumb suction control valve and keep it depressed while you set wall suction to the desired level.

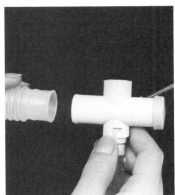

3 Connect the T-piece to the ventilator circuit. Make sure the irrigation port's closed.

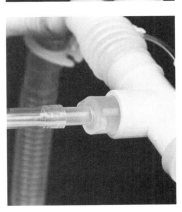

4 Attach the T-piece to the patient's endotracheal or tracheal tube.

Respiratory care

Using Trach Care closed suction system continued

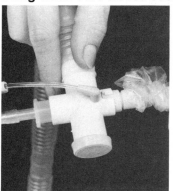

5 Gripping the T-piece with one hand, use the thumb and index finger of your other hand to carefully guide the catheter down the tube. (Leave the catheter in its protective wrapping.) *Important:* Keep the T-piece parallel with the patient's chin during this step.

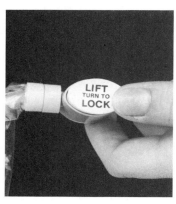

6 As needed, apply intermittent suction by depressing the thumb suction control valve.

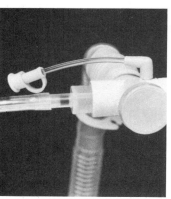

7 Still gripping the T-piece and depressing the suction control valve, gently withdraw the catheter to the catheter sleeve's fully extended length until you can see the black mark at the back of the T-piece.

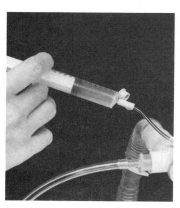

8 After suctioning, flush the catheter through the irrigation port. (Start suctioning before you begin flushing.) Flush slowly while you continue suction.
Finally, lift and turn the thumb piece 180° to the LOCK position.

The CyberSet speech system: Allowing intubated patients to speak

The doctor has just intubated your patient with an endotracheal (ET) tube. Because the tube makes speech impossible, your patient must rely on hand signals or an alphabet board to communicate—or you must read his lips. But these cumbersome methods often come up short, leaving him anxious, frustrated, and withdrawn. You worry, too, that you may miss something important because he can't adequately describe his symptoms.

This situation's all too familiar. But thanks to new technology, such as the CyberSet speech system featured here, it may someday become uncommon. Made by DACOMED Corporation, the system permits self-activated, easily understood speech, typically within minutes of the patient's first attempt. Indicated for any patient who needs an ET tube, it's especially useful for one who's likely to remain intubated for more than 24 hours.

The CyberSet speech system has two main components:
• a speaking ET (CyberSet) tube, with a main ventilating channel plus an extra lumen that conducts a speech tone to the posterior oral pharynx
• a voice generator, consisting of a pulse generator and a tone valve. To activate the hand-held, battery-operated pulse generator, the patient touches its membrane switch. The tone valve, which opens and closes by electrical impulses from the pulse generator, produces a tone when connected to a compressed gas source. The CyberSet tube conducts the generated tone to the oral pharynx; the patient uses his lips and tongue to shape the tone into words.

As the following photostory demonstrates, the CyberSet speech system is easy to set up and operate. Read on for details.

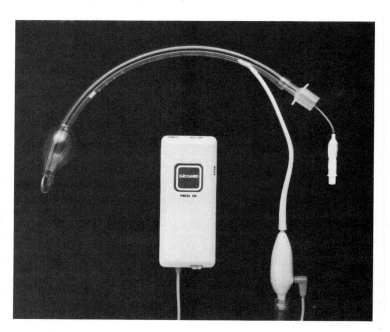

Setting up the CyberSet speech system

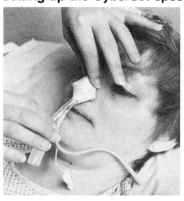

1 As needed, assist with intubation (nasal intubation produces the most intelligible speech). Then connect the oxygen tubing to a compressed gas source (air or oxygen) that's equipped with an adapter for the CyberSet tone valve. Make sure all connections are secure. *Note:* You'll place the patient on the ventilator, as ordered. For demonstration purposes, however, we haven't connected her tube to the ventilator.

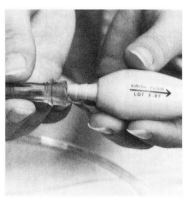

2 Run the oxygen tubing from the gas source to the "Christmas tree" valve on the tone valve, which is self-regulating.

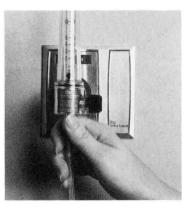

3 Let gas flow briefly, then check the flow meter; it should read zero.

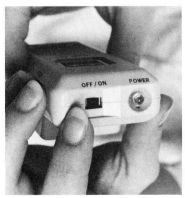

4 Connect the power cord from the pulse generator to the tone valve. Test the pulse generator by turning the OFF/ON switch to the ON position and pressing the membrane switch. The generator's lighted electronic display should flash and you should hear a tone; gas flows at 1 to 2 liters/minute.

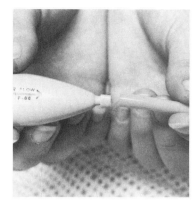

5 Connect the tone valve inlet to the CyberSet tube's tone inlet port, as the nurse is doing here.

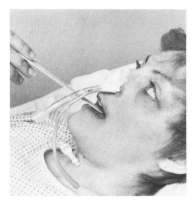

6 Check that the system's ready for use by activating the pulse generator, opening the patient's mouth, and depressing her tongue with a tongue depressor. You should hear a tone coming from her mouth.

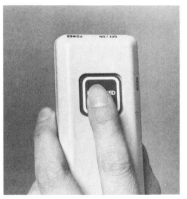

7 Instruct the patient to press the membrane switch (or, if necessary, the optional remote switch) while moving her lips to form words. Warn her that her voice will sound slightly artificial.

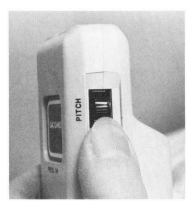

8 For best results, advise her to speak in short word groups; to exaggerate her mouth, lip, and tongue movements; and to adjust the pitch control dial (shown here) on the pulse generator to obtain the best pitch. If her speech sounds muffled or gurgled, periodically suction secretions from the CyberSet ports at her oral pharynx.

Respiratory care

Troubleshooting the CyberSet speech system

Use the chart below to help identify and deal with problems that can occur while your patient uses the CyberSet speech system.

Problem	Possible cause	Intervention
No tone from tone valve when patient activates voice generator	• Low battery power	• Check lighted electronic display on pulse generator; if it doesn't flash when activated, change battery.
	• Pulse generator improperly connected to tone valve	• Check connections to pulse generator and tone valve.
	• Tone valve improperly connected to gas source	• Check all connections and oxygen tubing.
	• Defective tone valve	• Replace tone valve.
	• Gas source not turned on	• Turn gas source to 50 psi.
	• Malfunction of remote switch (if used)	• Disconnect remote switch and activate pulse generator with membrane switch.
No tone audible from patient's mouth	• CyberSet ports blocked	• With cuff inflated, flush and then suction patient's oral pharynx, using a syringe connected to tone inlet.
	• Tone valve improperly connected	• Check airflow from tone valve. • Check oxygen tubing and all connections to tone valve.
Muffled speech	• Inadequate gas flow	• Set regulator to 50 psi and check all connections for leaks.
	• Excessive oral pharyngeal secretions	• Suction oral pharynx periodically.
	• Inadequate enunciation	• Instruct patient to exaggerate mouth, lip, and tongue movements.
	• Improperly adjusted pitch control	• Adjust pitch control to optimal level.

Nasal CPAP: Long-term treatment option for sleep apnea

Sleep apnea—episodic airflow cessation through the nose and mouth during sleep—can cause effects that range from merely annoying to severely disruptive. Traditional treatments—for example, tracheostomy and administration of antidepressants or respiratory stimulants—can cause serious adverse effects.

Now, a continuous positive airway pressure (CPAP) system suited for home or hospital use provides a comfortable, long-term treatment option with no reported adverse effects. It's indicated for patients with obstructive sleep apnea (caused by upper airway occlusion) or mixed sleep apnea (central breathing cessation followed by upper airway occlusion); central sleep apnea (cessation of respiratory muscle activity secondary to neurologic dysfunction) appears unresponsive to CPAP.

Researchers theorize that CPAP prevents apnea by splinting the pharyngeal area, thus reducing upper airway resistance and the amount of negative pressure needed to maintain airflow. Typically, CPAP treatment reduces the number of apneic episodes, improves oxygen saturation, and reduces diaphragmatic effort and upper airway muscle drive.

Shown at right, the SleepEasy II nasal CPAP system (Respironics Inc.) feeds pressurized air through a nasal mask that the patient wears as he sleeps. Because it covers only the nose, it permits mouth breathing if a power outage occurs. And because its flow generator doesn't exceed 20 cmH$_2$O, it doesn't subject the patient to dangerously high positive pressure if the valve becomes accidentally blocked.

The SleepEasy II system comes in two models—one for clinical use and one for home use. Before prescribing the home model for your patient, the doctor will order full-night diagnostic sleep studies to confirm obstructive or mixed sleep apnea and to determine the CPAP level needed to prevent apnea. To learn how to use the clinical model, read the photostory beginning on page 124. Then review the patient-teaching tips on page 125 to help your patient learn how to use the home model.

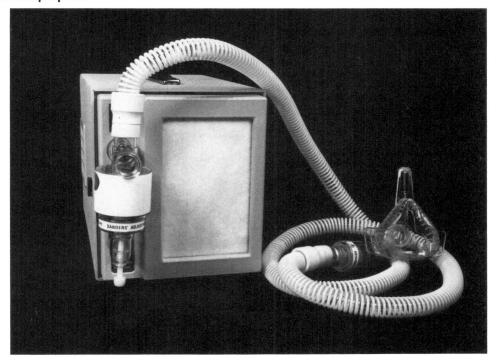

SleepEasy II nasal CPAP system
The SleepEasy II system includes a flow generator, a CPAP valve, an NRV-2 (nonrebreathing) valve, and a nasal mask. Other equipment components not shown here include additional tubing, a tubing coupler, and a plastic card with straps for securing the mask to the patient.

MINI-ASSESSMENT

Normal sleep and respiratory patterns

Each of two levels of sleep—non–rapid eye movement (NREM) and rapid eye movement (REM)—is associated with different ventilatory patterns. NREMs are subdivided into four stages:
• In *stage one*, a person feels drowsy. This transition between wakefulness and sleep lasts from 30 seconds to about 7 minutes. The respiratory pattern varies, possibly from shifts in CO$_2$ as the tidal volume decreases.
• In *stage two*, true sleep, the person's respirations seem regular, although apneas and hypopneas can occur.
• In *stages three* and *four*, referred to as delta sleep, apneas rarely occur.

REM sleep occurs approximately 90 minutes after a person enters NREM sleep. During REM, which lasts 10 to 20 minutes, neural activity increases; heart rate, blood pressure, and respiratory rate vary; and dreaming occurs. Skeletal muscle tone and intercostal activity diminish. Apneas also occur in this stage of sleep.

Normally, a person alternates between REM and NREM sleep. As the night progresses, REM periods lengthen and the person spends more NREM time in stage two and less in stages three and four. Occasionally, hypoxic arousal causes a person to reenter stage one. Normally, 30 apneas can occur in a 7-hour period of sleep.

Respiratory care

Setting up the SleepEasy II nasal CPAP system

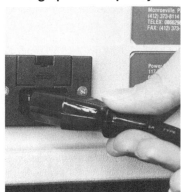

1 Insert the power cord into the input power receptacle on the flow generator's back, as the nurse is doing here. Then plug the cord into a 3-pronged outlet.

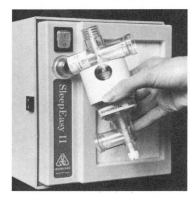

2 Connect the CPAP valve's inlet port to the flow generator's outlet adapter, as shown. Make sure the grooved port faces up.

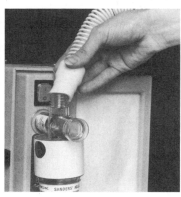

3 Attach one end of the tubing to the valve's grooved port. (If you need more tubing between the patient and the flow generator, use the tubing coupler to connect the additional piece of tubing.)

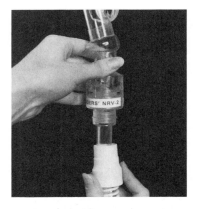

4 Connect the tubing's free end to the NRV-2 (nonrebreathing) valve's tubing-swivel end.

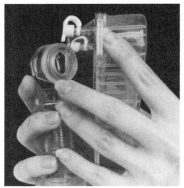

5 Prepare to attach the mask to the NRV-2 valve by removing the plastic split washer from the valve and pressing the valve into the back of the mask, as shown.

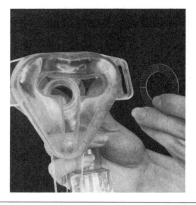

6 Take the plastic split washer (shown here) and pull it open slightly. Start it in the groove on the valve's neck and follow it around with a finger until it snaps in place. (To interrupt therapy, you can disassemble the NRV-2 between the valve and the swivel connector. During reassembly, make sure the closed wind deflector side of the NRV-2 is on the same side as the swivel connector's plastic washer.)

Applying the SleepEasy II mask

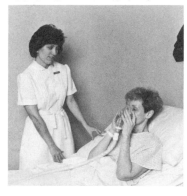

1 Teach the patient how to properly apply the nasal mask. First, ask her to hold the mask high on the bridge of her nose. To obtain a comfortable seal, have her spread the inner mask flaps and slide the mask down. *Important:* Make sure the mask (available in five sizes) fits the patient's face. The medium size fits a typical adult, so try it first.

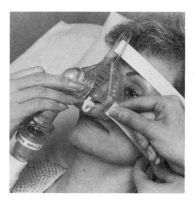

2 A plastic card with straps secures the mask. Position the plastic card behind the head, so the top strap rests high on the back of the head. (Make sure the straps lie between the card and the patient's head.) Feed the straps through the corresponding slots on the mask, with the Velcro fasteners away from the face; then stick the fasteners to the strap. (Don't tighten the straps yet.)

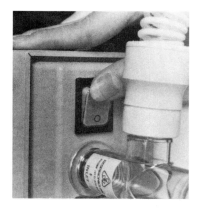

3 Tell the patient to keep her mouth closed. Then turn on the flow generator.

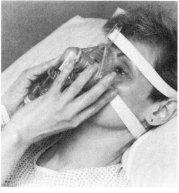

4 Now, have her gently press on the mask until she eliminates all air leaks around the cushion. Tell her that she needn't press hard.

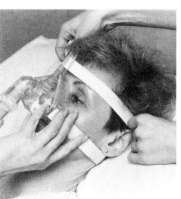

5 Next, adjust the upper strap to stabilize the mask and headgear. Then tighten the side straps until you eliminate leaks. Properly adjusted, straps should be snug, yet allow comfortable head movement in all directions. If leaks develop when the patient moves her head, readjust the straps; if they persist, try a different mask size.

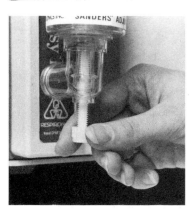

6 Now you're ready to use the system. First, make sure the adjustable CPAP valve opens freely and that air doesn't leak around the bridge of the nose. Set the CPAP valve at the lowest level, as shown, and let the patient sleep.

If she has an apneic episode, wake her and slightly increase the CPAP level, as ordered. Repeat the process until apneic episodes stop. Document the final, effective CPAP level; she'll use this level at home.

PATIENT TEACHING

When your patient's using a home nasal CPAP system

If your patient will use the SleepEasy II nasal CPAP system to treat sleep apnea, teach him how to use the home unit. Similar to the clinical unit shown on the preceding pages, it has fewer parts and a fixed (not adjustable) CPAP valve. Make sure he has a copy of the patient manual, and review it with him.

While teaching him about the system, explain that he may need 2 to 4 weeks to really feel comfortable with the equipment. He can relieve the sensation of too much pressure, common among patients just starting to use the equipment, by keeping his mouth shut before and during sleep.

Also emphasize these points:
• Call the doctor if symptoms of obstructive sleep apnea (daytime sleepiness, mood changes) recur. You may need a pressure adjustment.
• Make sure the mask fits snugly, without leaks. Leaks near your nose could irritate your eyes.
• After determining the proper fit for your mask and headgear, mark the straps with indelible ink or safety pins, so you needn't refit the mask every night.
• If your nose feels dry during treatment, try placing a humidifier about 8 feet from the flow generator's filter.
• If you develop a sinus problem or ear infection, temporarily discontinue treatment and call your doctor.
• Clean and care for the equipment as directed by the patient manual. Replace the intake filter as recommended—a dirty filter reduces airflow and lowers inspiration pressure, thus negating the therapy's benefits.
• If your face gets red around the mask, try loosening the straps a bit. (But remember, don't allow air leaks.) If the redness persists, you may need another size mask. Or, you may be having an allergic reaction to the mask. Your doctor may suggest that you apply a barrier under the mask.

Respiratory care

Introducing high-frequency jet ventilation

Your patient, an accident victim with head and chest injuries, needs mechanical ventilation. Because high-pressure ventilation could create undesirable chest wall movement, the doctor turns to high-frequency jet ventilation (HFJV).

HFJV employs a narrow injector cannula to deliver short, rapid bursts of oxygen to the airways under low pressure (see illustration). This combination of high rate, low tidal volumes, and low pressure enhances alveolar gas exchange without elevating peak inspiratory pressures and compromising cardiac output—the chief drawbacks of conventional high-volume, high-pressure mechanical ventilation.

Originally developed for a few specific situations that contraindicate conventional mechanical ventilation, HFJV now has new emergency applications. Because the cannula can be inserted directly into the trachea after cricothyrotomy, HFJV is useful when upper airway trauma prevents intubation. During CPR, it permits continuous ventilation during chest compression. And in patients with chest trauma, it minimizes chest wall movement.

You probably won't be responsible for setting up HFJV equipment, like Healthdyne's Impulse jet ventilator. However, because you may be responsible for monitoring a patient who's using it, familiarize yourself with its controls and alarms by examining the photo on the opposite page. *Important:* Read the manufacturer's manual and complete a training course before you attempt to operate the Impulse jet ventilator.

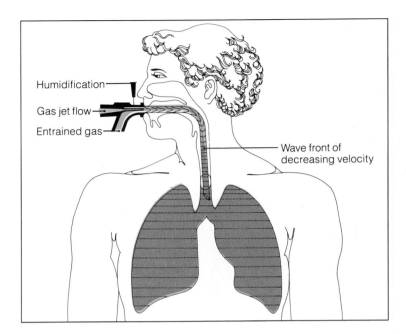

Humidification

Gas jet flow

Entrained gas

Wave front of decreasing velocity

TROUBLESHOOTING

The Impulse ventilator: Problem-solving tips

If the Impulse ventilator malfunctions, or if you hear or see an alarm, first check the patient to make sure he's adequately ventilated. Then proceed with troubleshooting. The following information suggests ways to solve a few potential problems.

Problem
Jet obstruction; jet pulses and continuous flow cease
Interventions
• Look for kinks and other obstructions in the jet line.
• Disconnect the jet line; if the alarm stops, reconnect the line.
• If the alarm doesn't stop when you disconnect the jet line, the alarm has malfunctioned.
• Make sure the jet delivery system—the catheter or endotracheal tube—is unobstructed and large enough to handle the flow.

Problem
Low inlet pressure
Interventions
• Check the air/nitrous oxide/oxygen pressure; it should be set at 50 psig.
• Check gas hoses for kinks or obstructions.
• Make sure you're using a high-flow blender, as recommended by the manufacturer.

Problem
Power loss
Interventions
• Check the power cord.
• Check for power failure.
• Replace the ventilator fuse, if necessary.
• Replace or recharge the battery, if necessary.

Problem
Low airway pressure
Interventions
• Determine whether the patient's condition has changed.
• Check all hoses, circuits, and water traps for leaks and loose connections.

Problem
High-pressure alarm sounds; jet temporarily stops pulsing
Interventions
• Check the patient—coughing or grunting can trigger this alarm. The alarm condition should self-correct and reset; the jet resumes automatically.
• If the alarm condition doesn't self-correct, check the expiratory circuit, airway sensing line, and endotracheal tube (or other patient delivery system) for obstructions.

Impulse jet ventilator

Low and high cmH₂O thumbwheel switches and indicators. Establish alarm setpoints from 0 to 99 cmH₂O. Jet pulse and airflow stops when high alarm goes off. The LOW ALARM DELAY knob and LOW ALARM AUDIO DELAY button delay the sounding and lighting of the low alarm.

Drive pressure control and display. Adjusts the jet's force from 0 to 60 psig; displays the pressure digitally.

%I-time control and display. Determines the breathing cycle percentage devoted to inspiration (I); digitally displays the percentage (ranging from 1% to 50%).

Power switch. In the ON (illuminated) position, supplies power to the ventilator.

Power loss indicator. Lights up and sounds an alarm when electric power to the ventilator drops below 90 to 95 v AC or eight v DC.

Minimum inspiration and maximum inspiration indicators. Light up when rate and %I time settings result in inspiratory time less than 10 milliseconds or more than 3 seconds.

Low inlet pressure indicator. Lights up when supply of gas pressure to the ventilator drops below 20 psig. (The ventilator will continue to operate.)

Jet obstruction indicator. Lights up when the jet line pressure doesn't fall below 50 cmH₂O after each pulse; shuts off the jet until the situation is corrected.

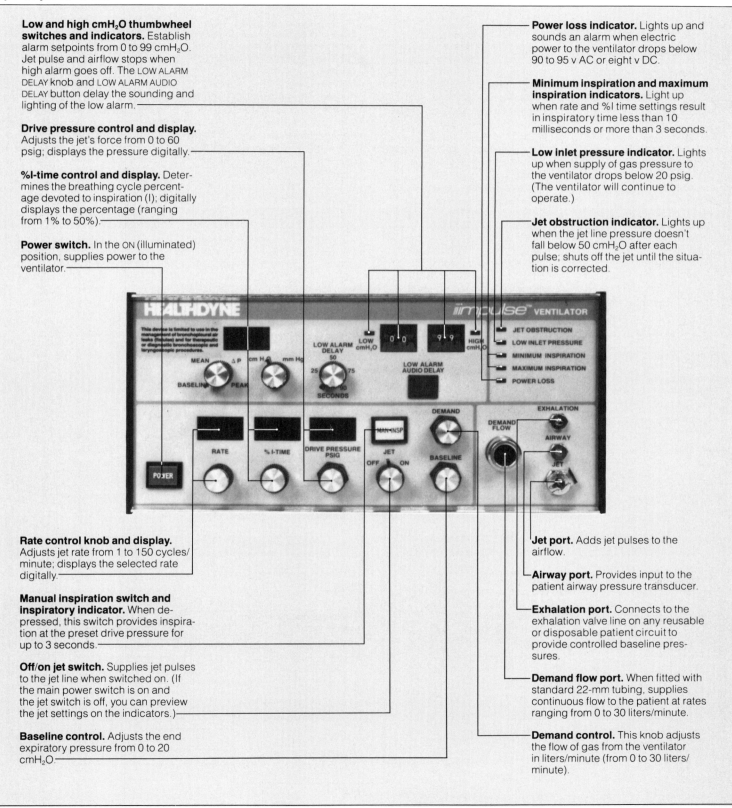

Rate control knob and display. Adjusts jet rate from 1 to 150 cycles/ minute; displays the selected rate digitally.

Manual inspiration switch and inspiratory indicator. When depressed, this switch provides inspiration at the preset drive pressure for up to 3 seconds.

Off/on jet switch. Supplies jet pulses to the jet line when switched on. (If the main power switch is on and the jet switch is off, you can preview the jet settings on the indicators.)

Baseline control. Adjusts the end expiratory pressure from 0 to 20 cmH₂O.

Jet port. Adds jet pulses to the airflow.

Airway port. Provides input to the patient airway pressure transducer.

Exhalation port. Connects to the exhalation valve line on any reusable or disposable patient circuit to provide controlled baseline pressures.

Demand flow port. When fitted with standard 22-mm tubing, supplies continuous flow to the patient at rates ranging from 0 to 30 liters/minute.

Demand control. This knob adjusts the flow of gas from the ventilator in liters/minute (from 0 to 30 liters/ minute).

Respiratory care

Learning about the Puritan-Bennett 7200 Microprocessor Ventilator

Sally Thomas, a 30-year-old teacher injured in an auto accident, is admitted to the intensive care unit with multiple injuries, including a flail chest. Her paradoxical chest movements and blood gases indicate that she's in acute respiratory distress. She's intubated and placed on a ventilator.

For patients like Ms. Thomas, the Puritan-Bennett 7200 Microprocessor Ventilator, featured here, provides precision respiratory support. With its computerized electronic circuit design, this equipment controls all ventilator functions and monitors patient and ventilator performance. Endowed with an extensive memory, the microprocessor can respond to operator-selected instructions or switch to its special memory, which activates

the emergency or backup systems. It also supplies the operator with digital readouts of performance data. If the system loses its DC power supply, a backup battery system retains ventilator settings for an hour. When stored, the special memory remains intact for 200 days.

How it works
To understand how this ventilator functions, review the diagram shown below. Note that the microprocessor integrates information to and from all of the system's components. When the operator inputs desired functions on the keyboard, sensors and valves in the pneumatic system activate the electronic circuits to adjust gas, flow, mix, and temperature. The patient service system delivers the oxygen/air

mix to the patient and returns the exhaled air to the ventilator. Finally, the display panel receives programming messages and data. Keep in mind that if faulty operating conditions occur, the computer's special memory overrides the operator-controlled one.

Safety features
The 7200 Microprocessor Ventilator senses faulty operating conditions quickly and alerts the operator to them. Its safety systems include:
• self-diagnostic tests. Performed before and during operation, these tests tell the operator whether the ventilator is functional. If it detects an error, the ventilator goes into backup ventilator mode until the problem is corrected.

• emergency ventilation modes. The ventilator activates one of four safety modes when it detects a system error. In *apnea ventilation, disconnect ventilation,* and *backup ventilator,* the ventilator continues to operate, using factory-preset parameters. In *safety-valve open,* the patient breathes room air and the ventilator shuts off.
• alarm system. Instead of a single alarm, the ventilator uses a hierarchy of alarms to signal problems. After one of the 12 alarms in the keyboard's ventilator status section sounds, the microprocessor monitors the situation and automatically resets the alarm if the situation self-corrects. See the chart on page 130 for details about some common alarm conditions.

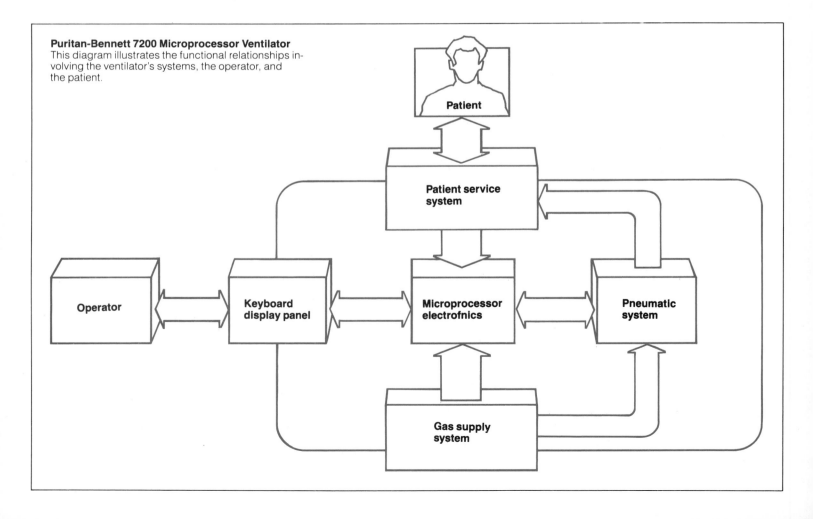

Puritan-Bennett 7200 Microprocessor Ventilator
This diagram illustrates the functional relationships involving the ventilator's systems, the operator, and the patient.

A closer look at the keyboard display panel

Setting up the 7200 Microprocessor Ventilator may not be a nursing responsibility in your hospital. But you should become familiar with the keyboard display panel so you can interpret data and respond to alarms. As shown below, the display panel has three basic sections:

• *Ventilator settings.* Allows the operator to set the ventilator according to the doctor's orders. This section includes the numerical keyboard; the message display screen; and settings for ventilation modes, waveforms, and mandatory respiratory parameters. The alarm threshold keys permit the operator to set limits for patient and ventilator performance.

• *Patient data.* Reflects the patient's response to the ventilator.

• *Ventilator status.* Indicates ventilator performance. For a quick assessment, check for blue (normal function), red (alarm situation), or yellow (alarm situation corrected) lights on the left-hand side. To identify specific problems, observe the 12 alarm indicators on the right-hand side.

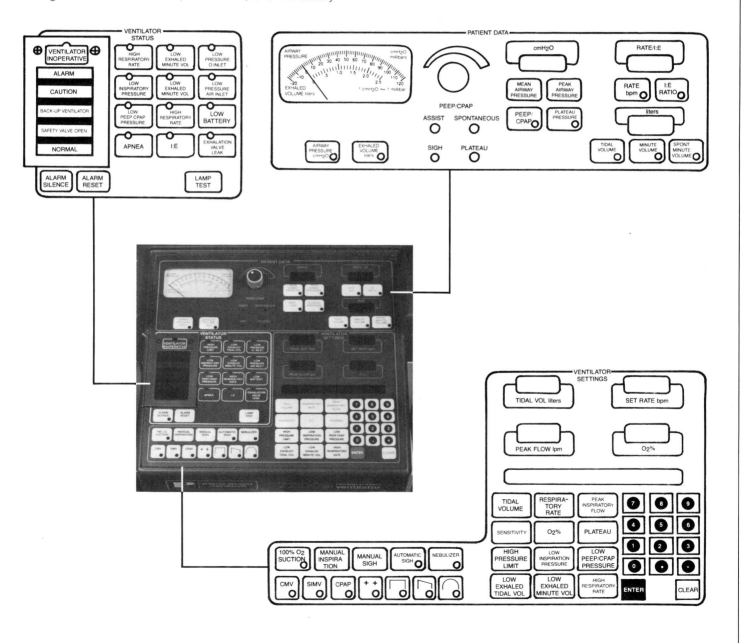

Respiratory care

Alarm and reset conditions: Some examples

Each of the 7200 Microprocessor Ventilator's 12 alarms will automatically reset under certain circumstances. This chart summarizes alarm and reset conditions for some of the ventilator's alarms.

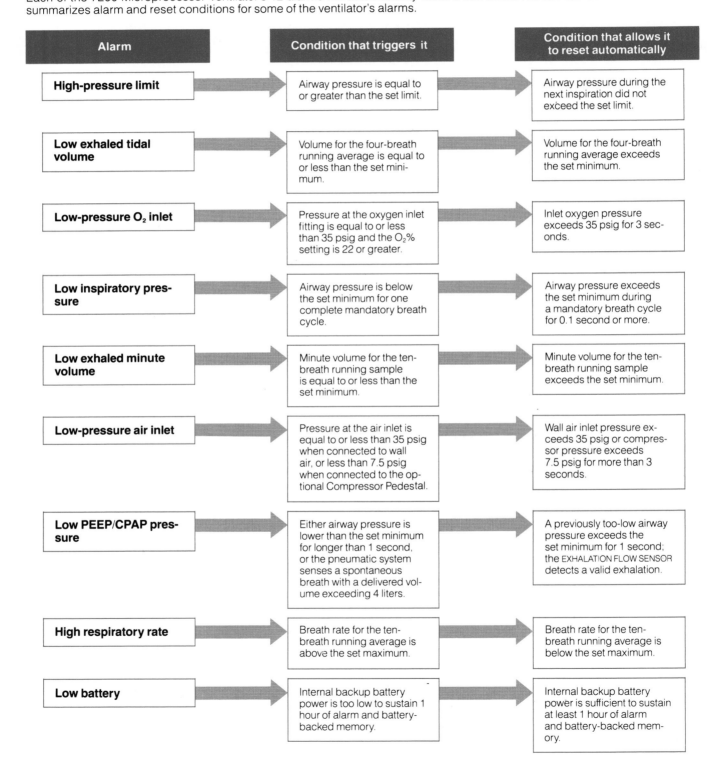

Alarm	Condition that triggers it	Condition that allows it to reset automatically
High-pressure limit	Airway pressure is equal to or greater than the set limit.	Airway pressure during the next inspiration did not exceed the set limit.
Low exhaled tidal volume	Volume for the four-breath running average is equal to or less than the set minimum.	Volume for the four-breath running average exceeds the set minimum.
Low-pressure O₂ inlet	Pressure at the oxygen inlet fitting is equal to or less than 35 psig and the O₂% setting is 22 or greater.	Inlet oxygen pressure exceeds 35 psig for 3 seconds.
Low inspiratory pressure	Airway pressure is below the set minimum for one complete mandatory breath cycle.	Airway pressure exceeds the set minimum during a mandatory breath cycle for 0.1 second or more.
Low exhaled minute volume	Minute volume for the ten-breath running sample is equal to or less than the set minimum.	Minute volume for the ten-breath running sample exceeds the set minimum.
Low-pressure air inlet	Pressure at the air inlet is equal to or less than 35 psig when connected to wall air, or less than 7.5 psig when connected to the optional Compressor Pedestal.	Wall air inlet pressure exceeds 35 psig or compressor pressure exceeds 7.5 psig for more than 3 seconds.
Low PEEP/CPAP pressure	Either airway pressure is lower than the set minimum for longer than 1 second, or the pneumatic system senses a spontaneous breath with a delivered volume exceeding 4 liters.	A previously too-low airway pressure exceeds the set minimum for 1 second; the EXHALATION FLOW SENSOR detects a valid exhalation.
High respiratory rate	Breath rate for the ten-breath running average is above the set maximum.	Breath rate for the ten-breath running average is below the set maximum.
Low battery	Internal backup battery power is too low to sustain 1 hour of alarm and battery-backed memory.	Internal backup battery power is sufficient to sustain at least 1 hour of alarm and battery-backed memory.

Neurologic care

If you're caring for a child with increased intracranial pressure, the doctor may order hyperventilation to achieve lower PaCO$_2$ levels. In this section, we familiarize you with this therapeutic option.

In addition, you'll learn about:
• therapeutic plasma exchange, now used to treat some neurologic disorders
• central pontine myelinolysis, a recently identified complication of rapid I.V. saline infusions
• a cervical collar that provides maximum stability for a patient who's suffered a neck injury.

Hyperventilation: Lowering PaCO$_2$ levels in children with increased ICP

If you care for a child with increased intracranial pressure (ICP), you may treat the problem by administering hyperventilation, as ordered. The most effective short-term means of reducing increased ICP, hyperventilation increases the rate and depth of a child's respiration, thus decreasing PaCO$_2$ levels. Falling PaCO$_2$ levels trigger vasoconstriction, which reduces cerebral blood flow (CBF); the decrease in intracranial blood volume lowers ICP.

Of course, this strategy poses an obvious risk: if CBF diminishes too much, the brain becomes ischemic.

Lowering PaCO$_2$ levels: How far?

Unfortunately, no one can say for sure how far you can safely lower PaCO$_2$ levels before ischemia develops. Some doctors favor reducing them between 30 and 35 mm Hg; others believe they can go as low as 20 mm Hg. And some doctors don't advocate any set lower limit.

In practice, you may see a child's PaCO$_2$ levels fall as low as 15 mm Hg during hyperventilation treatment, with a corresponding drop in ICP. However, this reduction in PaCO$_2$ levels occurs in association with other therapies (for example, ventricular drainage, barbi-

turate coma, or hypothermia), not in isolation. Monitor CBF closely throughout treatment.

Nursing considerations

You can manage hyperventilation in two ways: with mechanical ventilation or with manual ventilation—preferably by endotracheal tube, not mask. Manual ventilation can effectively reduce transient ICP increases.

If you're assisting with mechanical hyperventilation, follow these guidelines:
• Administer a barbiturate and a neuromuscular blocker—for example, thiopental sodium and pancuronium bromide (Pavulon)—as ordered. The barbiturate reduces cerebral metabolic requirements, which in turn reduces CBF and lowers ICP. The neuromuscular blocker prevents gastrointestinal reflux and makes intubation easier by paralyzing the child and allowing better visualization of the trachea. During therapy, a continuous Pavulon infusion prevents the child from fighting the ventilator, promoting passive hyperventilation and a large tidal volume.
• Throughout therapy, closely monitor arterial blood gas levels to ensure that PaCO$_2$ levels remain in the ordered range and that cerebral oxygenation is adequate.

SPECIAL CONSIDERATIONS

Recognizing increased ICP: Pediatric considerations

When assessing an infant or child for increased ICP, watch for lethargy, irritability, anorexia or poor feeding, vomiting, and (if increased ICP is persistent or chronic) cranial suture separation. Differences in cranial anatomy and the ability to communicate explain why other assessment findings vary according to the patient's age. See the list below for other telltale signs of increased ICP. Note: Use the Glasgow Coma Scale (see page 30) to assess a child's level of consciousness.

In infants:
• tense, bulging anterior fontanelle
• high-pitched cry
• increased head circumference (may be absent if increased ICP is acute)

• delayed or absent motor skills.

In children:
• headache
• diplopia or blurred vision
• nausea or vomiting
• papilledema (after 48 hours)
• seizures.

Late signs in infants and children:
• altered level of consciousness
• pupil dilation (unilateral or bilateral); sluggish response to light
• tachycardia, then bradycardia
• systolic hypertension
• widened pulse pressure
• altered respiratory rate and pattern
• apnea.

Neurologic care

Therapeutic plasma exchange: Neurologic applications

Also called plasmapheresis, therapeutic plasma exchange (TPE) removes unwanted substances—toxins, metabolic wastes, and plasma constituents implicated in disease—from the blood. Using TPE to treat neurologic disorders remains controversial: researchers have conflicting opinions about its effectiveness in recent clinical trials involving several neurologic disorders. However, TPE's ability to remove immunologically active substances from the blood suggests that it's a promising therapy for a limited number of neurologic diseases.

Because TPE's effects appear to be short-lived, it may be most useful against disorders of limited duration, such as Guillain-Barré syndrome. But it may also provide effective short-term treatment for some chronic disorders, such as multiple sclerosis and myasthenia gravis.

The illustration below shows how a TPE system works.

Nursing considerations
Only professionals trained to perform apheresis procedures should perform TPE. Your role may include monitoring vital signs and laboratory test results before, during, and after the procedure.

In addition, monitor the patient closely for signs and symptoms of potential complications, which include:
- red blood cell hemolysis
- citrate-induced hypocalcemia
- allergic reaction
- hemorrhage (secondary to anticoagulant administration)
- clotting problems
- fluid imbalance
- infection (from replacement fluids containing plasma).

How TPE works
The diagram below shows how the Therapore primary system (Sarns, Inc./3M) separates plasma from cellular components. After separation, cellular components mix with replacement fluid and return to the patient. Built-in safety features help ensure maximum plasma flow and optimum separation efficiencies without hemolysis, platelet loss, or complement activation.

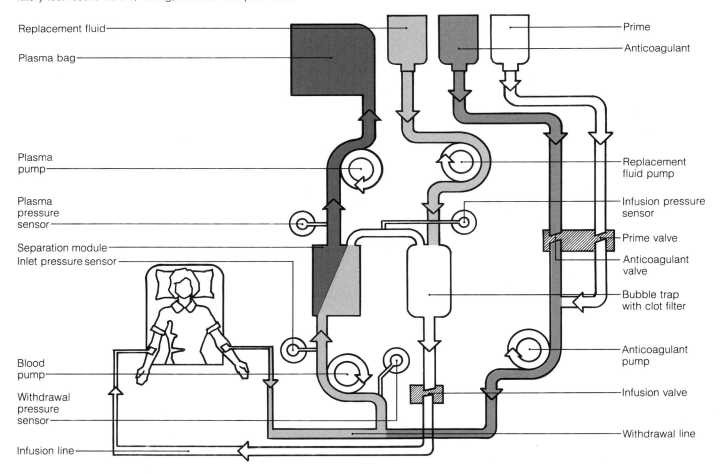

Applying Nec Loc

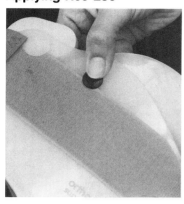

1 If your patient has a cervical spine injury, you may use the two-piece Nec Loc, shown here, to provide maximum stability. Prepare to apply the front portion by locking the black buttons in place, creating a chin rest.

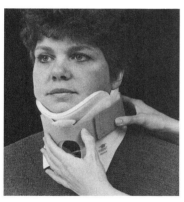

2 Then apply the front portion, as shown here. Wrap the orange strap behind the patient's neck, and secure it by pressing the tab against the Velcro strip on the Nec Loc's front.

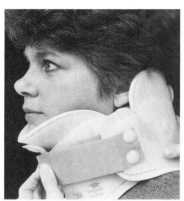

3 Apply the back portion and secure the orange strips to maintain proper immobilization.

Danger: Central pontine myelinolysis

Rapid infusion of an I.V. saline solution to correct fluid volume deficiencies—long a standard practice in emergency departments—has been linked to the development of central pontine myelinolysis (CPM) in some patients. Marked by pontine myelin destruction and disruption of the pyramidal tract, CPM causes severe, sometimes fatal, neurologic impairment. Patients with a severe electrolyte disturbance, particularly hyponatremia (serum sodium level less than 130 mEq/liter), are especially susceptible. The primary predisposing factors are malnutrition and alcoholism; others include chronic renal failure, hepatic disease, advanced cancer, acute hemorrhagic pancreatitis, and severe bacterial infections.

Typical clinical features of CPM include:
* nystagmus and palsies of cranial nerve VI, which restrict lateral eye movement
* altered level of consciousness, sometimes with pseudocoma or "locked in" syndrome
* pseudobulbar palsy, evidenced by dysarthrias and dysphagia
* quadriparesis.

Many of these mental and ocular changes resemble those found in acute thiamine (vitamin B_1) deficiency or Wernicke's encephalopathy; in fact, CPM and Wernicke's encephalopathy may coexist in the same patient.

If any patient—especially one suffering from malnutrition and/or alcoholism—develops these signs and symptoms, suspect CPM and notify the doctor immediately. Expect to administer thiamine (50 to 100 mg, either I.V. or I.M.). Perform frequent neurologic checks, as ordered, and monitor trends in serum sodium level. The doctor may order diagnostic studies, such as computed tomography scanning, magnetic resonance imaging, and brain stem and somatosensory evoked potentials.

To help prevent CPM, provide fluid and electrolyte replacement judiciously to volume-depleted patients, and avoid hypertonic saline solutions unless absolutely necessary.

Renal care

Simple and efficient, continuous arteriovenous hemofiltration (CAVH) has become an increasingly popular way to treat acute renal failure and fluid overload in many patients. By mimicking normal glomerular function, the process efficiently extracts plasma, water, and solutes at low pressures and low blood flow rates.

The Renaflo Advanced Hemofiltration System we're featuring here is designed for use in intensive care units. You may find yourself responsible for using it in the future—if you're not using it already.

Read the following pages to learn about the principles behind CAVH and its advantages and disadvantages. We also cover:
• setting up the Renaflo system and initiating treatment
• monitoring the patient throughout treatment
• troubleshooting problems
• discontinuing treatment.

Treating renal failure with continuous hemofiltration

Charles Jackson, a 69-year-old retired carpenter, underwent coronary artery bypass surgery 3 days ago. Within the past 24 hours, he has become oliguric and has developed renal failure. To treat the problem, his doctor has ordered continuous arteriovenous hemofiltration (CAVH), an alternative to hemodialysis and peritoneal dialysis that removes wastes without using dialysate.

If you're an ICU nurse, you may perform this procedure. To familiarize you with it, we'll feature the Renaflo Advanced Hemofiltration System on the following pages. To understand how it works, first review the principles behind CAVH.

What's CAVH?

A simpler system than hemodialysis, CAVH removes blood from the patient via an arterial line and filters it through a hemofilter, which removes water, electrolytes, and nonprotein-bound solutes at 400 to 800 ml/hour. These filtered substances, called the ultrafiltrate, drain into a collection container. Blood containing proteins and other molecules too large to be filtered return to the patient via a venous line. To benefit from CAVH, the patient needs good vascular access, preferably with a femoral catheter or Scribner shunt.

Fluid dynamic principles explain how CAVH works. If hydrostatic pressure exceeds oncotic pressure, fluid leaves the vascular space. The greater the pressure gradient, the greater the fluid removal. In CAVH, the patient's systolic blood pressure provides the hydrostatic pressure that propels blood through the filter. The ultrafiltrate line provides additional pressure, pulling ultrafiltrate into the ultrafiltrate compartment. For the system to continue working, these pressures must remain higher than pressure exerted by the plasma proteins—the oncotic pressure.

To ensure that CAVH works, you must:
• maintain blood flow between 50 and 100 ml/minute
• maintain systolic blood pressure above 60 mm Hg
• position the hemofilter at or below the patient's heart
• use an ultrafiltrate line that's at least 18″ long
• position the ultrafiltrate collection container on the floor
• keep the system heparinized.

CAVH's advantages

CAVH is typically performed for 2 to 10 days, 24 hours a day. Because CAVH employs less complex equipment than hemodialysis, it requires fewer skilled people to operate it. And its continuous, gradual action makes it ideal for hemodynamically unstable patients—

with CAVH, they experience less drastic fluid shifts and electrolyte imbalances than they would with either hemodialysis or peritoneal dialysis. Anuric patients receiving hyperalimentation infusions have a lower risk of fluid overload with CAVH's efficient fluid removal.

Patients who benefit from CAVH include those with:
• refractory congestive heart failure and pulmonary edema.
• acute renal failure.
• oliguria requiring large-volume fluid replacement.
• conditions causing chronic fluid overload, such as ascites and nephrotic syndrome.

Problems and precautions

As with any extracorporeal circulation system, CAVH can cause such problems as hemorrhage, clotting, fluid and electrolyte imbalances, and infection. You can minimize these risks with close monitoring and prompt intervention.

CAVH also filters out drugs, except for those that are protein-bound. Closely monitor the patient to maintain therapeutic drug levels.

To minimize clotting risks in the extracorporeal system, inject a 1,000 to 2,000 IU heparin bolus into the venous vascular access 2 to 3 minutes before treatment begins, as ordered. During treatment, maintain a continuous I.V. heparin infusion through the heparin infusion line on the arterial side.

To avoid bleeding problems, monitor clotting times throughout treatment. If bleeding problems develop, you can administer regional heparinization by giving heparin through the arterial line, then neutralizing the heparin before it reaches the patient by injecting protamine sulfate into the venous port.

To minimize the risk of hypovolemia and electrolyte imbalances, administer replacement fluids through the arterial or venous fluid administration lines, as ordered.

Variations

The Renaflo system featured on the next few pages can accommodate classic CAVH as well as all the variations, including:
• slow continuous ultrafiltration (SCUF). Indicated for patients with chronic conditions who don't need rapid blood filtration, SCUF removes filtrate at a slower rate: 150 to 300 ml/hour. Most patients undergoing SCUF don't need fluid replacement therapy.
• continuous arteriovenous hemodialysis (CAVHD) for enhanced urea and creatinine clearance. A dialyzing solution given through an ultrafiltration port provides the concentration gradient to remove these protein solutes by diffusion.

Renaflo Advanced Hemofiltration System: A closer look

As shown below, Minntech's Renaflo equipment includes a compact hemofilter encased in a plastic cylinder. Made up of several thousand polysulfone hollow fibers, the hemofilter acts as a semipermeable membrane that permits high filtration rates with minimal pressure fluctuations. This feature minimizes clotting in the filter, extending its period of usefulness.

As you see, the hemofilter has two side ports. You use only one to administer continuous arteriovenous hemofiltration (CAVH); you use both to administer continuous arteriovenous hemodialysis (CAVHD).

The filter attaches securely to the arterial, venous, and ultrafiltration lines with twist-lock and Luer-Lok connectors. The arterial line contains the heparin infusion line and a predilution fluid administration line to which a three-way stopcock is attached. The venous line has two postdilution infusion ports, which you can also use for regional heparinization and intravenous hyperalimentation. Both the arterial and venous lines also contain blood sampling ports.

The ultrafiltration line connects to the ultrafiltrate collection container (or to a suction device, if indicated).

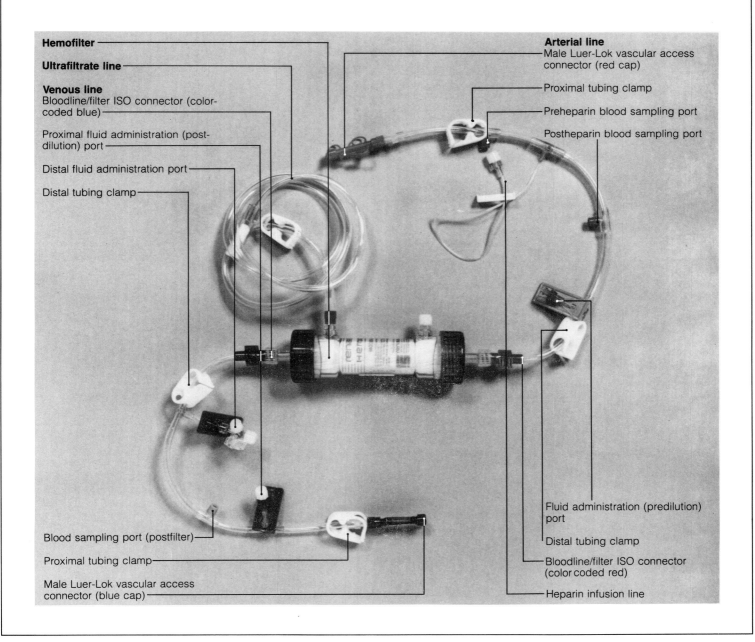

Renal care

How to set up the Renaflo system

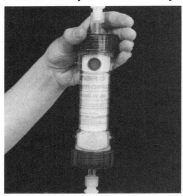

1 Besides the equipment supplied by the manufacturer, obtain a sterile graduated collection container, such as a urine collection bag, to hold the ultrafiltrate.

Wash your hands and maintain aseptic technique when-ever you open the system. Remove the Renaflo hemofilter (shown here) and blood tubing from the packages. Examine them for damage, and make sure all ports and connections are capped.

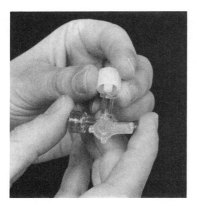

2 Open the pouch containing the two stopcocks and four Luer caps. Attach the Luer caps to the Luer connectors on the stopcocks, as shown in this photo.

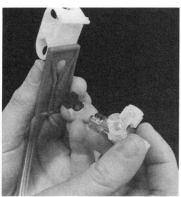

3 Remove and discard the Luer cap from the arterial tubing fluid administration (pre-dilution) port. Attach a stopcock to this port and tighten it. In the same manner, connect a stopcock to the distal venous fluid administration port.

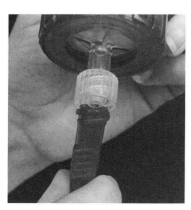

4 Now you're ready to connect the arterial line to the hemo-filter. Locate the International Standards Organization (ISO) connector on the arterial tubing, then the hemofilter's red inlet port. Remove and discard the end caps. Attach the arterial line to the filter port and tighten it clockwise.

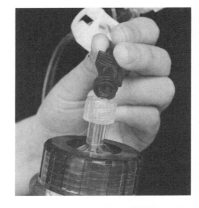

5 Use the same procedure to connect the blue venous tubing ISO connector to the filter's venous ISO connector.

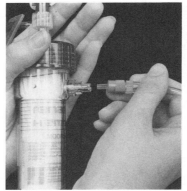

6 To connect the ultrafiltrate line to the hemofilter, remove the ultrafiltrate line's end cap by twisting the blue locking ring. Discard the cap. Remove and discard the blue cap from the ul-trafiltrate port proximal to the venous end of the hemofilter. Attach the ultrafiltrate line to this port, as shown. Tighten the locking ring. (Don't remove the white Luer cap from the ultrafil-trate port near the filter's arterial end. Use this port *only* for CAVHD.)

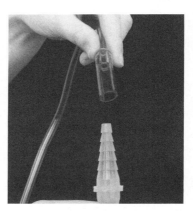

7 Remove the foam plug from the ultrafiltrate line, and attach the line to a graduated collection container.

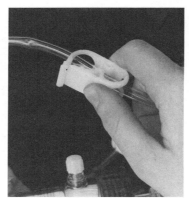

8 Close the five ratchet clamps on the arterial, venous, and ultrafiltrate tubing. Now that you've created a closed system, you're ready to begin priming. Read the next photo-story to learn how. *Caution:* Remember to use aseptic tech-nique whenever you open the system.

Priming the Renaflo system

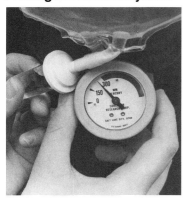

1 To prime the hemofilter and tubing, you need standard I.V. tubing; an I.V. pole; a large, sterile collection basin; and 2 liters of normal saline I.V. solution with 2,000 to 5,000 IU heparin added to each liter (as ordered).

Attach the I.V. tubing to 1 liter of heparinized saline solution. For rapid priming, attach a blood administration bag with a pressure cuff to the I.V. container and inflate to 300 mm Hg.

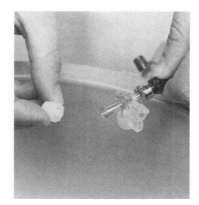

5 Before priming the arterial fluid administration line and stopcock, remove the Luer caps from the stopcock. Allow fluid to fill the stopcock. Then close the slide clamp and replace the Luer caps.

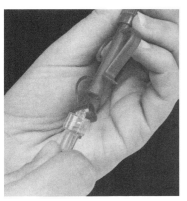

2 Locate the red rinse connector on the arterial tubing. Open its cap and insert the I.V. tubing.

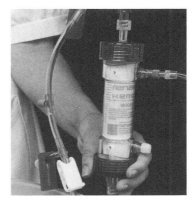

6 You're now ready to prime the hemofilter. Position the filter vertically, with the arterial inlet port pointing down.

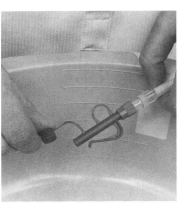

3 Open the blue rinse connector cap on the venous tubing. Secure this tubing to a sterile collection basin that's large enough to collect the priming solution after it rinses the system (see photo). *Important:* Maintain sterility whenever you open the system.

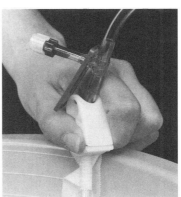

7 Open the distal arterial tubing clamp (nearest the filter) and the proximal and distal venous tubing clamps. Continue to hold the filter vertically.

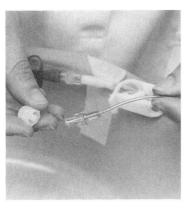

4 To prime the heparin infusion line, open the proximal arterial tubing clamp (nearest the patient) and the I.V. tubing. Hold the heparin line over the basin, remove the Luer cap, and prime the line until air disappears. Clamp the heparin line and replace the Luer cap.

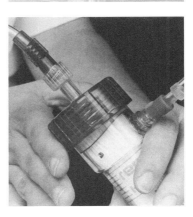

8 Begin infusing the I.V. solution through the hemofilter. Gently rock the filter while tapping the blue header nut with your fingers.

Renal care

Priming the Renaflow system continued

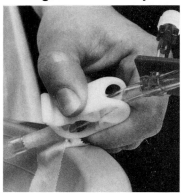

9 When the first liter of I.V. solution has infused, close both venous tubing clamps and the I.V. tubing clamp. Remove and discard the empty I.V. container. Empty the collection basin, if necessary.

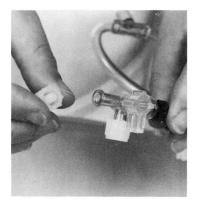

13 Now unclamp the distal venous tubing (nearest the hemofilter), and infuse fluid into the distal venous fluid administration line and stopcock. Repeat the procedure you followed to prime the arterial fluid administration line. Close the slide clamp.

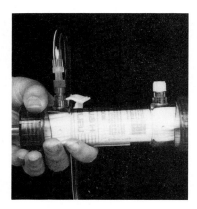

10 Attach the second container of heparinized I.V. solution to the I.V. tubing. To prime the ultrafiltrate line and compartment, position the hemofilter horizontally, with the ultrafiltrate ports pointing upward, as shown here.

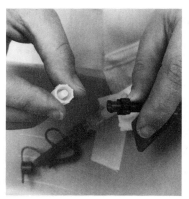

14 Prime the proximal venous fluid administration line, close the slide clamp, and replace the cap.

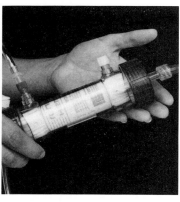

11 Next, open the ultrafiltrate and I.V. tubing clamps. To facilitate air removal, gently rock and tap the filter.

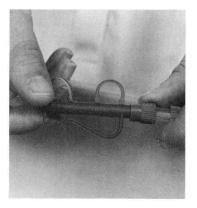

15 Finish priming by opening the proximal venous clamp (nearest the basin). Clear air from the line. When only 50 ml of solution remains in the I.V. container, close all clamps. Remove the I.V. container and the I.V. tubing. Close the venous and arterial rinse caps.
  Recheck the system, making sure clamps and tubing are attached securely.

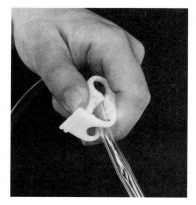

12 Rinse the ultrafiltrate compartment with 500 ml of I.V. solution; then clamp the ultrafiltrate line.

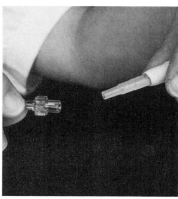

16 Now that you've primed the system, attach the ordered I.V. heparin solution to the heparin infusion line; you can also attach I.V. replacement fluid to the predilution or postdilution port (as ordered). Read the following photostory for details on initiating treatment.

Initiating treatment with Renaflo

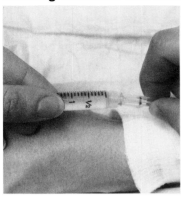

1 Before connecting the patient to the hemofilter, examine his vascular access for bleeding or clotting. If he has femoral catheters in place, make sure they're secure. Administer a heparin loading dose (if ordered) into the venous vascular access and allow the heparin to circulate 2 to 3 minutes before initiating blood flow.

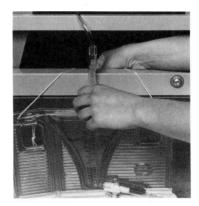

5 Place the ultrafiltration collection container below the hemofilter. To establish good blood flow, keep the ultrafiltrate tubing clamped for 3 to 5 minutes while blood flows through the filter.

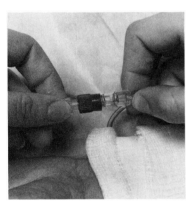

2 Then attach the arterial tubing to his arterial access and the venous tubing to his venous access. Remove his access clamps.

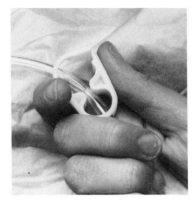

6 Open the ultrafiltrate clamp to begin the ultrafiltrate flow. To maximize negative pressure in the ultrafiltrate compartment, maintain a continuous column of fluid in the ultrafiltrate line.

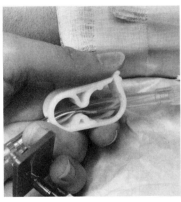

3 To begin CAVH, first open both venous tubing clamps, then the arterial clamp nearest the hemofilter, and finally the arterial clamp nearest the patient. You should see blood begin to flow through the hemofilter.

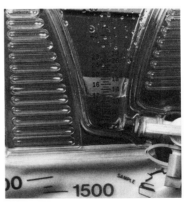

7 Obtain a baseline ultrafiltration rate (UFR) by measuring UFR for 1 minute.

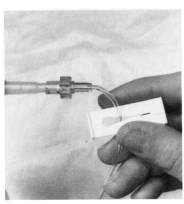

4 Open the slide clamp on the heparin infusion line and begin the heparin infusion at the prescribed rate.

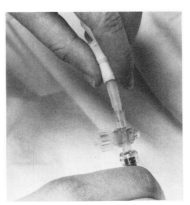

8 Administer replacement fluids through the arterial (predilution) or the venous (postdilution) port, as ordered. Monitor the patient's vital signs. Frequently check all lines and the filter connections for leaks and kinks.

Renal care

Discontinuing treatment

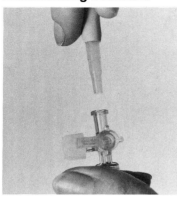

1 Attach I.V. tubing from a 500-ml bag of normal saline solution to the three-way stopcock on the arterial fluid administration port.

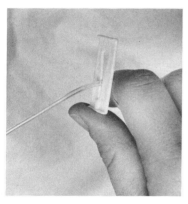

2 Stop the heparin and replacement infusions on the venous and arterial lines.

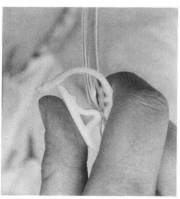

3 Clamp the ultrafiltrate tubing.

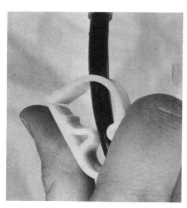

4 Close the proximal arterial clamp (nearest the patient) and clamp the arterial venous access.

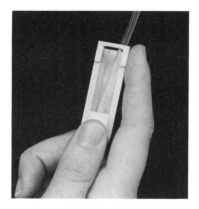

5 To return blood in the hemofilter to the patient, open the I.V. clamp and infuse the saline solution until blood clears from the venous line.

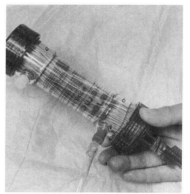

6 For rapid clearance, position the venous outlet lower than the arterial inlet.

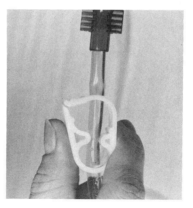

7 Then close the venous clamps and the distal arterial clamp (nearest the filter). Clamp the venous vascular access.

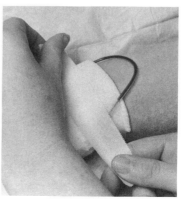

8 If the patient has an arteriovenous shunt, reconnect it. If he has femoral catheters in place, remove them (if ordered) and apply manual pressure. Then apply a dressing to the site.
  Discard the hemofilter and other disposable equipment. Wash your hands.

Caring for a patient on CAVH: Your role

Easily implemented, continuous arteriovenous hemofiltration (CAVH) has become increasingly popular. With training and supervision, many ICU nurses now assemble the equipment, carry out the procedure, and monitor the patient. In some hospitals, a dialysis nurse prepares the patient's venous access and initiates treatment; she also serves as the primary resource for troubleshooting problems.

If you're caring for a patient who needs CAVH, explain the procedure to him and his family, and answer their questions. Tell them that you'll monitor his condition closely throughout treatment. Obtain baseline assessment measurements: vital signs, weight, and cardiac output.

In addition, you have the following responsibilities.

Monitoring the patient
● Establish baseline electrolyte, pH, serum protein, and hematocrit values before therapy begins.
● Obtain vital sign measurements (including central venous pressure and pulmonary artery wedge pressure measurements) every 15 minutes during the first hour of treatment and every 4 hours thereafter. Report any significant changes.
● Monitor the ultrafiltration rate (UFR). If the rate changes by more than 20%, notify the doctor.
● Record fluid intake and output hourly.
● Obtain clotting times (activated clotting time or partial thromboplastin time) every 4 hours. Adjust the heparin and protamine dosage, as ordered.
● Obtain specimens for arterial blood gas measurements and filtrate chemistries, as ordered.
● Obtain specimens for serum electrolyte and hematocrit measurements, as ordered (usually every 4 to 6 hours).
⬛ *Nursing tip:* If you're using postdilution replacement fluid, ultrafiltrate has approximately the same electrolyte composition as plasma. If permitted, you can collect specimens from the ultrafiltrate chamber and avoid subjecting the patient to repeated venipunctures.
● Monitor the patient for fluid and electrolyte imbalance and replace fluids according to his hourly fluid loss, as ordered. Calculate output (ultrafiltrate plus urine output, gastrointestinal losses, and other drainage) and intake (for example, nasogastric feedings and I.V. infusions); then titrate replacement volume as indicated.
● Infuse the ordered replacement fluid (usually a modified saline solution supplemented with calcium or magnesium and acetate, lactate, or bicarbonate) through either the pre- or postdilution port. (Using the predilution port increases the filtration rate, but it's more costly.)
● Closely monitor a severely catabolic patient to maintain adequate nutrition and to avoid fluid and electrolyte imbalance. Such a patient may require as much as 3 to 5 liters of intravenous hyperalimentation daily. You can supply this level of nutrition with CAVH, providing his ultrafiltrate output remains high and you replace lost electrolytes.
● Check pulses distal to arterial access sites.
● Watch for bleeding.

Monitoring the system
● Keep extra clamps and shunt connectors at the bedside.
● Check lines every hour for cracks, kinks, leaks, and loose connections.
● Assess for clotting. If it develops, the UFR drops and dark streaks appear in the arterial blood.
● If you suspect clotting, you may need to change the filter or increase the heparin dosage, as ordered.
● Look for blood in the ultrafiltrate collection container, which indicates capillary leaks in the filter. Clamp the ultrafiltrate line, notify the doctor, and prepare to change the filter.

Organ donation

Demand for organs and tissues continues to far outweigh the supply. Every day, thousands of people wait for word that a heart, kidney, or liver has been found for them. For these patients, organ donation can prolong life.

As a nurse, you help identify potential donors. You may also be responsible for maintaining organ and tissue viability before the harvesting procedure.

Organ and tissue donation: Preserving viability

If you're caring for a potential donor, notify the organ procurement agency affiliated with your hospital as soon as possible. Or call the North American Transplant Coordinators Organization's 24-hour hotline for emergency help (1-800-24-DONOR).

Be prepared to supply the organ procurement coordinator with the potential donor's admission date, diagnosis, blood pressure, urinary output, and ABO blood group. A transplant coordinator will conduct a detailed medical evaluation. The transplant surgeon ultimately decides whether to accept organs for transplant.

Maintain aseptic technique for all invasive procedures, to prevent sepsis. Also obtain a blood specimen for an HIV (human immunodeficiency virus) antibody test. Potential donors are now routinely screened for evidence of infection by HIV, which causes acquired immune deficiency syndrome (AIDS). The following chart details other nursing considerations, according to donated organ.

In general, cancer and infection involving the donor tissue at the time of death preclude donation. However, cancer isn't necessarily a contraindication for corneal donation.

ORGANS

KIDNEY
For patients with end-stage renal disease
Nursing considerations
• The donor should be between ages 1 and 60.
• Contraindications include prolonged untreated hypertension and renal disease.
• Maintain the donor's vital functions.
• Document fluid intake and output. Assess urine for amount, color, and odor.
• Monitor urine osmolality.
• Monitor serum electrolytes and maintain fluid and electrolyte balance.
• Monitor creatinine and blood urea nitrogen levels.
• Obtain specimens for urinalysis and for culture and sensitivity.

LIVER
For patients with end-stage liver disease, with a life expectancy of 1 year or less
Nursing considerations
• The donor should be between ages 6 months and 50 years.
• Prepare the donor for liver function studies, as ordered.
• Maintain vital functions.

HEART
For patients with end-stage heart disease
Nursing considerations
• A male donor should be younger than age 35; a female donor should be younger than age 40.
• Maintain the donor's vital functions.
• Obtain a 12-lead EKG.
• Initiate continuous cardiac monitoring.
• Measure blood pressure at least hourly.
• Document fluid intake and output.
• Obtain specimens for cardiac enzyme studies.

HEART AND LUNG
For patients with end-stage heart disease and pulmonary complications
Nursing considerations
• The donor should be between ages 1 and 50.
• Maintain the donor's vital functions.
• Obtain a 12-lead EKG and initiate continuous cardiac monitoring.
• Obtain specimens for cardiac enzyme studies.
• Monitor arterial blood gas values.
• Assess acid/base balance.

• Monitor pulmonary status by assessing breath sounds, chest expansion, and sputum production and quality. Watch for circumoral cyanosis and subcutaneous emphysema.
• Monitor fluid intake and output.
• Obtain specimens for sputum Gram stain and for culture and sensitivity.

PANCREAS
For patients with long-term insulin-dependent diabetes who have diabetic complications
Nursing considerations
• The donor should be between ages 14 and 45.
• Maintain the donor's vital functions.

TISSUES

BONE
For patients needing spinal fusion or neurosurgical repair
Nursing considerations
• The donor should be between ages 15 and 70. (Younger potential donors may be considered individually.)
• Tissue should be removed within 6 to 12 hours of death if the body isn't refrigerated; within 24 hours with refrigeration.

SKIN
For patients with extensive third-degree burns
Nursing considerations
• The donor should be between ages 15 and 75.
• Skin should be removed within 30 hours (with refrigeration).
• Inspect for color, temperature, texture and turgor; and for lesions and edema.
• Reposition the donor frequently. Protect skin integrity with such protective devices as sheepskin or an egg-crate mattress.

CORNEA
For patients with corneal disease or damage
Nursing considerations
• The donor should be younger than age 90.
• Inspect the eye for injury, infection, and other abnormalities. Note scleral color.
• Keep the donor's eyelids closed to prevent corneal abrasion.
• Administer ophthalmic medications, as ordered.
• The eye should be removed within 6 hours of death.

Caring for the
Special Patient

Obstetrics

Gynecology

Pediatrics

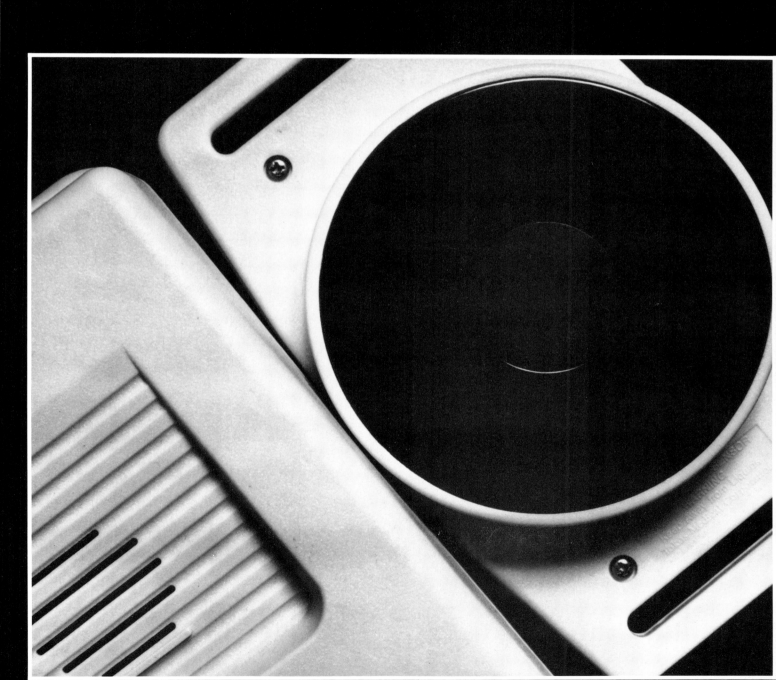

Obstetrics

For many patients, recent advances in obstetrics have improved the chances for successful pregnancy, labor, and delivery. In the following pages, you'll learn how to assess a pregnant patient's risk of preterm labor and recognize warning signs. You'll also learn how to intervene appropriately if preterm labor occurs.

For a patient at high risk, the doctor may prescribe TERM GUARD, a home monitoring device. Read about it on page 145.

In this section, we also discuss chorionic villi sampling, an increasingly popular alternative to amniocentesis for detecting fetal anomalies, and transcutaneous electrical nerve stimulation, which the doctor may prescribe for pain control during labor and delivery.

Preterm labor: Assessment and intervention guidelines

Defined as labor occurring after 20 weeks' but before 37 weeks' gestation, preterm labor can lead to preterm birth—the leading cause of infant death and disability. Diagnostic criteria for preterm labor include contractions less than 10 minutes apart plus at least one of the following:
• cervical dilation of 2 cm or more
• at least 75% cervical effacement
• progressive cervical changes during observation.

New approaches that include risk assessment programs, early identification, prompt medical treatment, and home uterine monitoring now prevent preterm labor's progression to preterm birth for many high-risk women.

Risk assessment
Although doctors haven't determined precisely what causes preterm labor, they've identified certain socioeconomic and medical risk factors. Socioeconomic factors include poverty, stress, and cigarette smoking. Women who perform heavy physical labor or stressful work or who commute more than 30 minutes to work also have a higher risk.

Medical risk factors include history of:
• premature labor
• spontaneous or induced abortions
• cervical conization
• pyelonephritis
• uterine anomaly
• diethylstilbestrol exposure
• two or more stillbirths or neonatal deaths
• cyanotic heart disease
• renal failure.
Pregnancy-related factors that increase the risk for preterm labor include multiple gestation, abdominal surgery during pregnancy, placenta previa, inappropriate weight gain, and uterine irritability.

Warning signs
Many women who go into preterm labor experience a prodromal stage lasting hours or even days before cervical dilation occurs. But if the woman's contractions aren't painful or if she has never experienced labor, she may not realize she's in labor. For this reason, all high-risk patients should know the warning signs of preterm labor:
• regular uterine contractions lasting more than 1 hour
• dull, low backache
• menstrual-like cramps
• feeling of pressure in the lower back, abdomen, or thighs
• intermittent pelvic pressure
• an increase or change in vaginal discharge (may be watery, slightly bloody, or mucous)
• premature membrane rupture
• intestinal cramping, possibly with diarrhea.

Intervention
Advise a woman who suspects preterm labor to drink two or three glasses of water or juice, rest on her left side, and palpate her uterus for contractions. She should call the doctor if symptoms don't subside within an hour, or if symptoms worsen.

Expect the doctor to order monitoring of uterine contractions for any woman admitted to the hospital for suspected preterm labor. Some women require only the most conservative treatment—hydration and bed rest.

Others may need labor-arresting drugs, such as ritodrine (Yutopar), terbutaline (Bricanyl), or magnesium sulfate. Because these drugs pose a significant risk to the mother, the doctor will assess maternal and fetal conditions carefully before deciding whether to order them. (Ritodrine or terbutaline shouldn't be given if the patient's pulse rate exceeds 140 beats/minute or if she's having trouble breathing.)

Note: These drugs are effective only with cervical dilation of less than 4 cm, so preterm labor must be identified soon after onset.

Home management
If labor has been successfully arrested, the patient may be managed at home on ritodrine or terbutaline and self-uterine palpation. Some patients may also use the TERM GUARD home monitor, an ambulatory uterine monitor that transmits data by telephone to a central station for analysis. This new device may detect labor early enough for effective drug therapy. For more information on TERM GUARD, see the following page.

Using TERM GUARD to detect uterine activity

Preterm labor, a leading cause of infant mortality, threatens as many as 10% of all pregnancies. Many of these threatened pregnancies could be prolonged if therapy were begun early.

TERM GUARD, a monitor that senses even subtle uterine contractions, is now being used to detect excessive uterine activity, which could indicate that labor has begun. Designed by Tokos Medical Corporation for ambulatory patients, the TERM GUARD system combines home uterine monitoring with perinatal nursing care. For many women at high risk of preterm labor and delivery, these services provide an alternative to hospitalization during the late stages of pregnancy.

How the TERM GUARD system works

As prescribed by her doctor, a high-risk patient begins using TERM GUARD (shown below) after the 20th week of pregnancy. First, she undergoes a training program. A Tokos perinatal nurse teaches her how to use the equipment, recognize signs and symptoms of preterm labor, and minimize risks. The nurse also reviews and reinforces the doctor's instructions. Tokos nurses remain available 24 hours a day, 7 days a week, to respond to questions or problems.

The patient uses TERM GUARD at home twice a day for an hour at a time. Using a lightweight belt, she wears the sensor on her abdomen. A small recorder carried in a shoulder strap records uterine contractions the sensor detects. This handy arrangement permits her to continue most routine daily activities during the monitoring period. (However, some patients are instructed to rest during this time).

At a prearranged time, a TERM GUARD nurse telephones. The patient then transmits data stored in the recorder by pressing the recorder's button and directing the recorder at her telephone receiver. The recorder transmits 2 hours of information in just 6 minutes.

If the transmitted data indicates an increase in the frequency and duration of uterine contractions, the nurse may instruct the patient to remonitor. Similarly, if the patient experiences unusual symptoms, she resumes monitoring and sends an emergency transmission to the TERM GUARD center. When a TERM GUARD nurse sees any indication of preterm labor, she notifies the doctor immediately.

Who benefits?

Indications for TERM GUARD include:
- previous preterm labor or delivery
- uterine irritability
- cervical dilation or effacement
- placenta previa
- polyhydramnios
- previous uterine surgery
- incompetent cervix
- large uterine fibroids
- pyelonephritis or recurrent urinary tract infection
- multiple gestation.

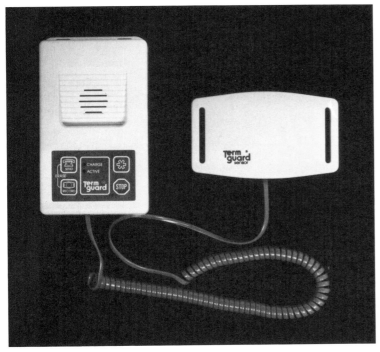

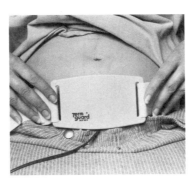

The patient positions the TERM GUARD sensor at the center of her abdomen below the umbilicus, as shown here.

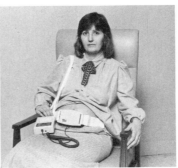

She wears the recorder on a shoulder strap, as this photo shows. During the monitoring period, this device records uterine contractions detected by the sensor.

Obstetrics

Chorionic villi sampling: An alternative to amniocentesis

An experimental prenatal test, chorionic villi sampling (CVS) may someday replace amniocentesis for quick, safe detection of fetal chromosomal and biochemical disorders. The procedure's performed during the first trimester of pregnancy. Preliminary results may be available within hours; complete results within a few days. In contrast, amniocentesis can't be performed before the 16th week of pregnancy, and the results aren't available for at least 2 weeks.

Chorionic villi—fingerlike projections surrounding the embryonic membrane—eventually give rise to the placenta. Cells obtained from a sample can reveal fetal disorders because these cells originate with the fetus, not the mother.

For best results, sampling should occur between the 8th and 10th weeks of pregnancy. Before 7 weeks, the villi cover the embryo and make selective sampling difficult. After 10 weeks, maternal cells begin to grow over the villi and the amniotic sac starts to fill the uterine cavity, making the procedure difficult and potentially dangerous.

To help the doctor collect a chorionic villi sample, place the patient in the lithotomy position. The doctor checks the patient's uterus placement bimanually, then inserts a speculum and swabs the cervix with an antiseptic solution. If necessary, he may use a tenaculum to straighten an acutely flexed uterus, permitting cannula insertion. Guided by ultrasound and possibly endoscopy, he directs a catheter through the cannula to the villi. Applying suction to the catheter, he then removes about 30 mg of tissue from the villi. After withdrawing the sample, he places it in a Petri dish for dissecting microscope examination. A portion of the sample's then cultured for further testing. Although the procedure doesn't require anesthesia, the patient may feel minor discomfort.

CVS results can be used to detect about 200 diseases. For instance, direct analysis of rapidly dividing fetal cells can detect chromosome disorders; DNA analysis can reveal hemoglobinopathies; and lysosomal enzyme assays can screen for lysosomal storage disorders, such as Tay-Sachs disease. Unlike amniocentesis, CVS *can't* detect complications in cases of Rh sensitization, identify neural tube defects (such as spina bifida), or determine pulmonary maturity.

CVS appears to provide reliable results except when the sample contains too few cells or the cells don't grow in culture. Like amniocentesis, the procedure carries a small risk of spontaneous abortion, cramps, infection, and bleeding.

Using TENS for obstetric analgesia

A familiar pain-relief option for surgical patients, transcutaneous electrical nerve stimulation (TENS) now has a new use: pain relief during labor and delivery. Safe and effective for many patients, TENS doesn't expose the mother and fetus to the hazards of drug therapy. Used with other pain-relief methods, such as body relaxation and breathing techniques, TENS provides a safe alternative to spinal anesthesia during vaginal delivery in patients at risk of uterine rupture. Unlike drug therapy, TENS won't mask severe uterine pain, a warning sign of impending rupture. TENS can also provide pain relief during delivery of the placenta and during the immediate postpartum period. For many patients, it also relieves postcesarean and episiotomy pain.

How does TENS work?

Through electrodes applied to the skin, a TENS unit transmits a mild electric current, which provides gentle local transcutaneous stimulation. The gate control theory of pain may explain why TENS works: its pulsed alternating current may prevent transmission of pain stimuli to the spinal cord. However, the placebo effect may also play a part.

To use TENS, the patient holds the stimulator device in her hand and increases or decreases stimulation as needed. Thus, she gains a sense of control over her pain. She may feel a mild tingling sensation during stimulation. Some patients experience local irritation under the electrodes.

Nursing considerations

• Teach the patient about TENS before labor begins, if possible.
• Initiate TENS therapy early in labor.
• Apply the electrodes near the sacral column.
• Let the patient regulate stimulation by herself, unless she becomes uncomfortable and asks for help.
• Support her during breathing and relaxation exercises.
Note: A TENS unit may interfere with electric fetal monitors. Try to minimize interference by reducing TENS amplitude.

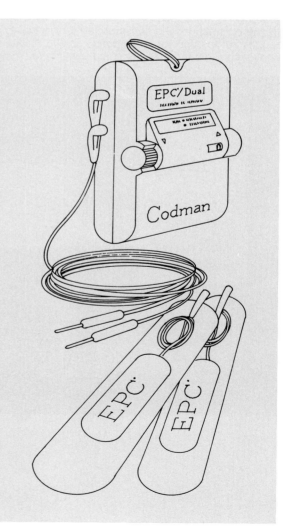

Gynecology

In the next few pages, we familiarize you with two new techniques aimed at early breast cancer detection. The MammaCare method of breast self-examination (BSE), which is more comprehensive than conventional BSE, trains women to locate breast lumps and distinguish potentially cancerous lumps from benign tissue. We provide a photostory that illustrates the MammaCare method beginning on page 148.

Breast transillumination can also detect breast cancer early. Capable of accurately identifying even small cancerous lumps, it uses harmless light rays—not X-rays—to produce diagnostic images.

You'll also find information on the contraceptive sponge and on newly developed techniques designed to help infertile women conceive. Read on for details.

UPDATE

MammaCare: A new approach to breast self-examination

Breast cancer strikes about 100,000 American women every year. Because women find most cancerous lumps themselves, breast self-examination (BSE) proves crucial to early cancer detection. Yet many women don't know how to perform BSE, and those who do may become discouraged by their inability to interpret the breast tissue variations they feel. Frustrated because they can't distinguish harmless breast nodules from potentially dangerous lumps, some even stop doing BSE.

To make BSE more useful, a University of Florida research team developed the MammaCare method—now offered at 25 authorized centers and, by special arrangement, through family doctors. MammaCare trains women to differentiate nodules from potentially cancerous lumps and to detect lumps as small as 5 mm in diameter (in contrast, the average lump found by women practicing other BSE methods measures about 38 mm).

Using various artificial breasts as training models, the MammaCare instructor teaches the patient an examination method that includes the following components:
- *skill training.* The patient learns to palpate her breasts using the flats, or pads, of her middle three fingers. Holding these fingers together, she moves them in a circular motion so that the circumference of the circle traced by her middle finger measures about 1 cm. This permits contact with tissue textures and contours that she might miss by pressing with her fingertips, as taught in conventional BSE methods.
- *discrimination training.* The patient learns to differentiate between large and small lumps, hard and soft lumps, and fixed and mobile lumps—and between each of these characteristics and normal nodular tissue.
- *pressure training.* The patient learns to use three different pressure levels to bring her fingers into contact with all potential lumps without pushing the lumps aside or concealing them in deeper tissue. At each spot she palpates, she makes three circles—first, using light pressure that barely moves the skin but would detect a tiny mobile lump just beneath the surface; next, pressing midway down into breast tissue; and finally, pressing hard, probing down to the ribs to detect any lump near the bone.
- *systematic search pattern.* The patient learns to examine her breasts in parallel vertical strips that cover all breast tissue—including the axilla and collarbone regions. To ensure thorough palpation, she overlaps along each vertical strip, then overlaps the strips.

After practicing these techniques on an artificial breast that closely matches her own breasts in nodularity and density, the patient examines her own breasts under the instructor's guidance. To evaluate the patient's detection skills, the instructor shines a light that casts a pattern of numbered boxes over the patient's chest, allowing the instructor to identify any areas that weren't palpated. She also teaches the patient how to examine her breasts visually for suspicious signs.

The patient keeps the artificial breast for 3 months for home practice. She also receives a calendar to remind her of monthly examination dates and a set of charts to document each month's findings. The instructor schedules a follow-up visit to make sure the patient retains her skills.

In the following photostory, we take you through a typical MammaCare instruction session. For more information on MammaCare—including how to become a MammaCare instructor—write to the Mammatech Corporation, 930 N.W. 8th Ave., Gainesville, Florida 32601; or call 1-800-MAM-CARE.

Gynecology

Teaching the MammaCare breast self-examination method

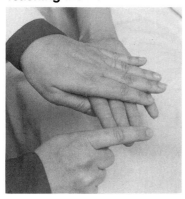

1 MammaCare instruction takes about an hour. You need special training from the Mammatech Corporation to teach the MammaCare method. For some basic instruction steps, read this photostory.

The MammaCare instructor explains the three-finger palpation technique (the patient presses on her breasts in a circular motion using the pads of her middle three fingers).

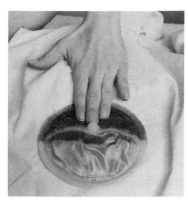

2 Next, the instructor shows the patient how to identify normal nodular breast tissue by palpating a nodule-containing artificial breast, which the patient places on her chest (see photo).

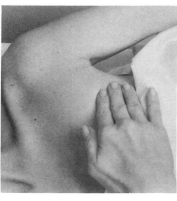

3 The patient then palpates her own breast in a region where the instructor has found nodules (usually the upper outer quadrant, as with the patient shown here).

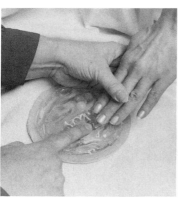

4 Using a special lump-discrimination artificial breast, the instructor explains how to differentiate lumps by size, hardness, depth, and mobility.

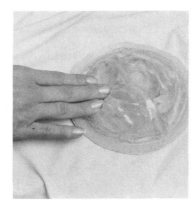

5 The patient then learns how to use light, medium, and deep pressure to palpate the breast. In this photo, the patient's using deep palpation to detect lumps near the base of the artificial breast.

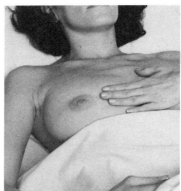

6 The instructor then tells the patient to palpate her own breast using all three pressure levels.

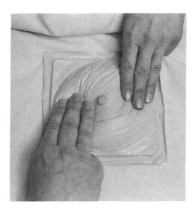

7 Now the instructor selects an artificial breast, like the one shown here, that closely matches the patient's breasts in density and nodularity.

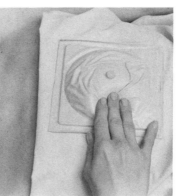

8 After explaining Mamma-Care's vertical-strip search pattern, the instructor tells the patient to examine the artificial breast in vertical strips.

CARING FOR THE SPECIAL PATIENT

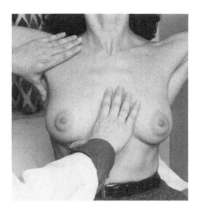

9 Before having the patient examine her own breasts, the instructor points out the boundaries of a complete breast examination.

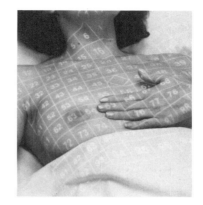

11 The instructor shines a Baum lamp on the patient's chest, as shown. While the patient examines her breasts, the instructor marks a paper grid that matches the Baum lamp's grid. This procedure lets the instructor identify unpalpated areas.

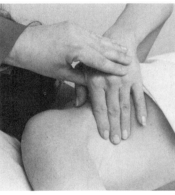

10 Placing the patient's hand on the outer boundary, the instructor tells the patient to begin her examination.

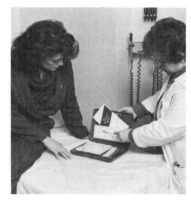

12 At the end of the training session, the instructor gives the patient the tissue-matched artificial breast and other materials to help her practice MammaCare confidently at home.

Transillumination: A new technique for breast assessment

Newly developed, transillumination (also called diaphanography or light scanning) provides diagnostic breast images without exposing the patient to X-rays. Here's how it works: light in the red and near-infrared range is projected through breast tissue and photographed by video camera. A computer then transforms the transmitted light, which is normally invisible to the human eye, into images on a video screen. Because of differences in tissue density, lesions and highly vascular areas (which may surround cancerous tumors) appear darker than normal tissue. The procedure also permits the doctor to compare both breasts for asymmetry, which suggests pathology.

Safe, quick, and painless, transillumination has obvious advantages for women who need regular breast exams but who fear the repeated X-ray exposure mammography requires. Because it's risk-free, young women can safely undergo routine examinations. It's also indicated for women with radiographically dense breasts, palpable lumps, and nipple discharge.

Research indicates that transillumination reliably identifies small tumors not detectable by ultrasound and helps the doctor to distinguish between malignant and benign tumors. It's currently an adjunct to mammography and other breast imaging techniques. In the near future, however, it may become an independent screening method.

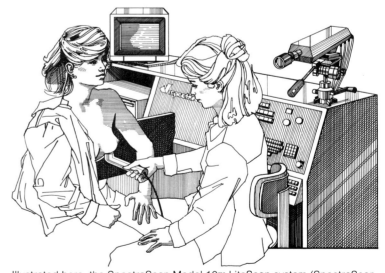

Illustrated here, the SpectraScan Model 10ms LiteScan system (SpectraScan, Inc.) has a special split-screen feature that allows the operator to make immediate bilateral comparisons; it can also provide side-by-side comparisons of serial examinations. As you can see, the operator can easily watch the video monitor as she works.

Gynecology

Today Contraceptive Sponge: Another birth control option

Your patient, who's age 36, has been taking birth control pills for almost 15 years. Although she's had no adverse effects, she's concerned about continuing to use birth control pills as she grows older. When she asks you about alternatives, you discuss the *Today* Contraceptive Sponge, shown below, as an option.

Available over the counter, the *Today* sponge offers an alternative to the pill, diaphragm, and condom. Unlike the pill, the sponge isn't associated with any serious side effects. Effective for a longer time than the diaphragm or condom, it's up to 91% effective when used correctly. Among reversible birth control methods, only the pill and the intrauterine device (no longer available in the United States) can claim higher success rates.

Three-way effectiveness

Made of polyurethane foam, the sponge contains nonoxynol-9, a widely used spermicide that's also available in many over-the-counter contraceptive foams. Thoroughly soaking the sponge with water before application releases the spermicide.

After application, the sponge prevents conception primarily by destroying sperm on contact. It also blocks the cervical entrance and absorbs sperm.

Because the sponge remains effective for 24 hours, a woman can have intercourse numerous times without reapplying a spermicide. She must leave the sponge in place for at least 6 hours after last having intercourse.

Thoroughly tested, the sponge causes no toxic effects and doesn't increase a woman's risk of toxic shock syndrome (TSS). (In fact, it may offer some protection against the bacteria that cause TSS.) However, some users have reported experiencing irritation or discomfort.

Patient teaching

Review the following illustrations for details on inserting and removing the sponge; then review them with your patient. If she has never used such a product before, reassure her that she'll become more adept at the procedure with practice.

If she has trouble removing the sponge, she's probably just tense. Suggest this relaxation technique:
• Tense abdominal and vaginal muscles completely for 5 seconds.
• Relax completely.
• Take a deep breath and bear down as though having a bowel movement; then remove the sponge.

For further information, your patient can call the toll-free *Today* Talkline, open 24 hours a day, 7 days a week: (800) 223-2329; in California, (800) 222-2329.

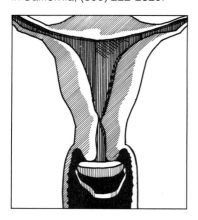

The sponge's depression fits over the cervix. The loop on the opposite side permits the woman to remove the sponge easily.

Inserting and removing the *Today* Contraceptive Sponge

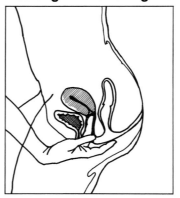

1 Give your patient the following instructions for inserting the *Today* sponge.
Squat and insert your middle finger as far as it will go. Gently feel for the cervix, which feels firm and round (like the end of your nose).

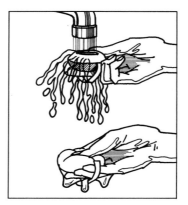

2 Prepare the sponge by thoroughly wetting it with clean tap water until it's soaked. Squeeze it gently—it should feel wet and soapy.
Then fold it in half, so the dimple faces up and the loop faces down.

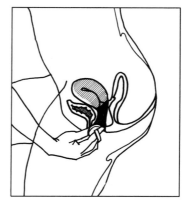

3 Bend your wrist, so you're pointing toward the vagina. Then squat slightly with your legs apart (or stand and raise one leg). Slide the sponge into the vagina, using one or two fingers.
Push the sponge deep into the vagina and put it over the cervix. Slide a finger around the sponge's edge to make sure the sponge covers the cervix.

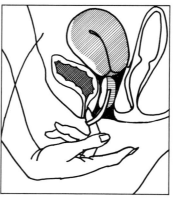

4 To remove the sponge, insert a finger into the vagina and reach up and back to find the sponge's loop. (If you can't find the loop, try bearing down with your abdominal muscles.) Hook your finger around the loop and pull out the sponge with a slow, gentle motion. (If you prefer, you can also remove the sponge by grasping it between two fingers.) *Remember:* Wait at least 6 hours after intercourse before removing the sponge.

Comparing infertility treatments

For pregnancy to occur, the male must have sufficient sperm of normal form and mobility that are capable of fertilizing an egg. The female must:
• ovulate
• have unobstructed, undamaged fallopian tubes
• have a uterine lining conducive to embryo implantation, growth, and development
• have sperm-receptive cervical mucus.

As recently as 20 years ago, fewer than 30% of infertile couples could be treated successfully. Today, an infertile couple has a 96.4% chance of conceiving a child. This dramatically improved success rate reflects technical advances and a new understanding of endocrinology and genetics, which has led to more effective ways to aid conception and support a pregnancy to term.

To compare common infertility treatments, study the chart below.

Treatment	Procedure	Special considerations
In vitro fertilization (IVF)	Male sperm and female eggs are placed together for fertilization outside the body; fertilized eggs are then transferred to uterus.	• Used mostly for couples with unexplained infertility
Gamete intrafallopian transfer	Abbreviated IVF procedure: sperm and eggs are placed immediately into fallopian tube(s) instead of being placed in culture media first.	• Less expensive than IVF because procedure's about 2 days shorter
Cryopreservation	Fertilized eggs are prepared and frozen for future implantation.	• Allows postponement of transfer until optimal uterine environment exists • Decreases multiple pregnancy risk and saves some fertilized eggs for future use by limiting the number of eggs transferred at one time
Intrauterine insemination	Sperm collected through masturbation are washed to remove seminal plasma, then inseminated directly into uterus during fertile period.	• Suitable for couples who have abnormal sperm count, poor postcoital tests, male or female sperm antibodies, poor cervical mucus, or unexplained infertility • Expensive and time-consuming (requires 1 hour preparation time; woman must remain in doctor's office up to 30 minutes after insemination to allow cervical mucus to seal over cervical os)
Laparoscopy	Doctor inserts laparoscope through umbilicus, then uses laser to treat endometriosis or repair damaged tube.	• Can usually be done on outpatient basis, reducing hospitalization time, recovery period, and risk of postoperative adhesion formation
Transcervical balloon tuboplasty	Doctor places balloon catheter into blocked fallopian tube via cervix, then inflates balloon to dilate tube and disperse obstructive fibrous tissue.	• Still experimental • Usually performed on outpatient basis • Costs much less than IVF or microsurgery

How the cervical cup aids conception

Artificial insemination has become an increasingly popular conception technique for infertile couples. The Milex **pro-ception** oligospermia cup shown below aids artificial insemination by holding sperm at the cervical os, thus maximizing the number of sperm that contact the cervical mucosa. The cup can aid homologous insemination (using the husband's sperm, rather than donor sperm) when anatomic anomalies, low sperm count, psychologically induced impotence, or a hostile cervical environment interferes with normal conception.

As the photograph shows, the cup has a hollow stem with a white ball inside. After the doctor places the cup on the woman's cervix and introduces sperm, he pushes the ball up the stem to prevent sperm from escaping.

To use the cup, a couple may follow this procedure to attempt homologous artificial insemination:
• The husband practices abstinence for 5 days before the wife's ovulation date. He and his wife then have intercourse while he wears a special polyethylene condom to collect sperm. (He shouldn't use a rubber condom because of its spermicidal properties.)
• As instructed by the doctor, the wife may use a special douche (such as **pro-ception** SPERM NUTRIENT) to create a favorable environment for sperm.
• The wife brings the sperm to the doctor's office as soon as possible after collection. The doctor may add penicillin to the semen to prevent bacterial growth.
• After aspirating the collected semen into a syringe via a polyethylene tubing attachment, the doctor fits an appropriately sized cup on the wife's cervix (the cup's available in 9 sizes).
• Next, he advances the syringe's tubing through the hole in the side of the cup's stem, until the tubing's tip reaches the cup. Then he injects the sperm into the cup.
• To prevent sperm from escaping, he uses a special tamper rod to push the stem's ball up to the cup. Finally, he folds the stem's end and pushes it into the loop.

As instructed, the woman removes the cup in 3 or 4 hours. (Because the cup prevents normal uterine drainage, leaving it in place longer than 12 hours may invite complications.) To remove it, she first loosens it with a finger to break suction. She then gently pulls the stem to extract the cup.

The cup may be reused by the same patient, provided it's first disinfected as recommended by the manufacturer.

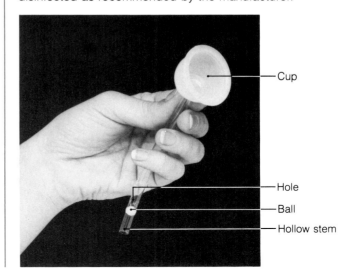

— Cup

— Hole

— Ball

— Hollow stem

Pediatrics

Infants and children always challenge your ingenuity and nursing skills. The following pages introduce you to some recent advances in pediatric care that will make your job easier while improving patient care.

For instance, consider the FirstTemp thermometer featured on these two pages. By measuring tympanic temperature, it provides an accurate reading of core body temperature—noninvasively.

Similarly, the Babe-Shade represents an advance for premature newborns, whose retinas may be damaged by ordinary nursery light. This simple device protects the infant's eyes without depriving him of sight or eye contact with those around him. Read about Babe-Shade on page 155.

We also acquaint you with two new drugs: ribavirin and somatrem.

Introducing FirstTemp: A noninvasive thermometer

Now you can accurately assess a sleeping infant's core body temperature without even awakening him. FirstTemp, the noninvasive thermometer shown below, instantly reveals your patient's temperature by electronically analyzing infrared energy given off by the tympanic membrane and ear canal. Because the tympanic membrane shares blood supply with the hypothalamus (the body's temperature regulator), tympanic membrane temperature closely correlates to core body temperature.

To use FirstTemp, simply occlude the ear canal's external opening with the probe tip, as shown in the following photostory. The digital display window shows the temperature (in either Centigrade or Fahrenheit) in less than 2 seconds.

Battery-operated, FirstTemp can take over 1,000 temperatures before it needs recharging; it automatically recalibrates when you replace the probe after each reading. Disposable probe covers guard against infection (an unlikely complication because skin, not a mucous membrane, lines the ear canal). Although especially practical for pediatric patients, FirstTemp works equally well with adults.

Temperature equivalents

While using the tympanic mode, you can program FirstTemp to display temperatures that approximate oral, rectal, or core temperature. For example, if your hospital also uses rectal thermometers, you may program FirstTemp to display the rectal temperature equivalent for consistency.

Surface scanning

At the press of a button, you can also convert FirstTemp to a surface-scanning instrument for assessing:
- skin temperature at a burn site
- vascular integrity in casted limbs
- wound healing rates
- incipient infection or infiltration at a venipuncture site.

Because the probe never touches the skin, you won't hurt the patient or contaminate a wound.

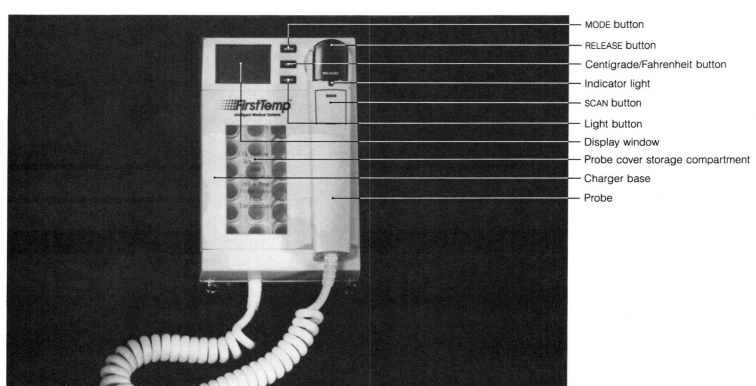

MODE button
RELEASE button
Centigrade/Fahrenheit button
Indicator light
SCAN button
Light button
Display window
Probe cover storage compartment
Charger base
Probe

Taking tympanic temperature with FirstTemp

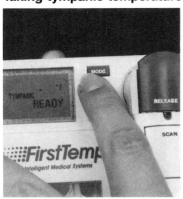

1 Remove FirstTemp from its charger base. If necessary, select the tympanic mode by pressing the MODE button. (Look for *TYMPANIC* in the display window.)

Wait for *READY* to appear in the window, as shown.

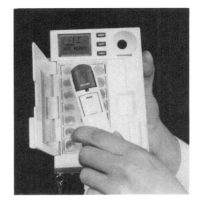

4 Open the probe cover storage compartment and press the probe into a disposable probe cover, as shown. (Press hard enough to detach the cover from its cassette.)

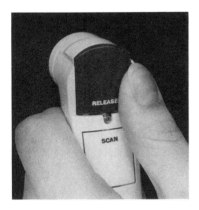

2 Press the blue RELEASE button and simultaneously lift the probe.

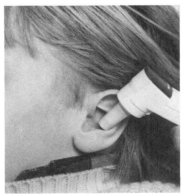

5 With the probe cover in place, insert the probe's tip into the external ear canal opening, just far enough to seal the opening (don't apply pressure). If an infant's ear is too small to accommodate the probe's tip, occlude the meatus and press *gently.* (For best results, try to prevent the child from moving his head during the procedure.)

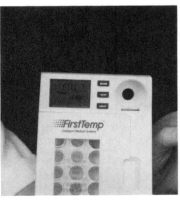

3 Check the window for temperature equivalent mode. You'll see one of these messages: *CAL* (factory calibration), *OrL* (oral temperature equivalent), *rEC* (rectal temperature equivalent), or *COr* (core temperature equivalent). If you want to change the temperature equivalent mode, follow the procedure described below.

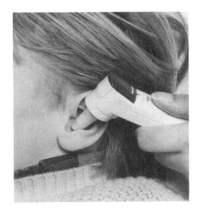

6 After positioning the probe, press the SCAN button on the probe handle, as shown, and wait 1 to 2 seconds: you'll hear intermittent beeping and see the probe's red light illuminate. Read the patient's temperature in the display window.

Remove the probe from the ear opening, press the RELEASE button to discard the probe cover, and replace the probe in its cradle. Replace FirstTemp on its charger base between uses.

Changing the temperature equivalent

Besides factory calibration, FirstTemp can display oral, rectal, or core temperature equivalents. If you want to change the temperature equivalent mode, simultaneously press the MODE and SCAN buttons. The window displays the current equivalence—for example, *OrL* (oral).

Each time you simultaneously press the MODE and SCAN buttons, the window advances to a new temperature equivalent mode. Continue the procedure until the mode you want appears—for example, *rEC* (rectal), as shown here. Press MODE to lock in the chosen equivalent mode.

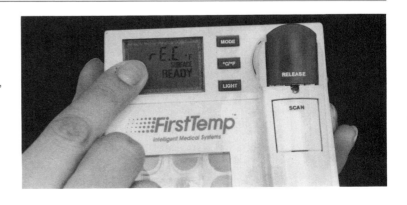

Pediatrics

Taking surface temperature with FirstTemp

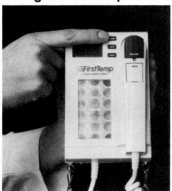

1 Remove FirstTemp from its charger base. If necessary, select surface mode by pressing the MODE button. Wait for *READY* to appear in the window.

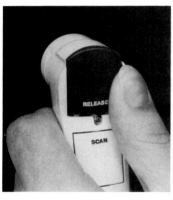

2 Press the RELEASE button and simultaneously lift the probe. Apply a disposable probe cover.

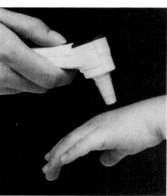

3 Hold the probe's tip no more than ½" above the area to be scanned, as shown here. Don't let the tip touch tissue.
Press the SCAN button. You'll hear a tone and see the temperature displayed in the window.

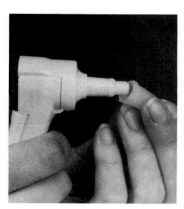

4 After completing the scan, release the SCAN button. Press the RELEASE button and discard the probe cover.
Replace the probe in its cradle. Keep FirstTemp on its charger base between uses.

Treating RSV infection with ribavirin

The single most important cause of bronchopneumonia, tracheo-bronchitis, and pneumonia in infants and young children, respiratory syncytial virus (RSV) is a major cause of fatal respiratory disease in the first year of life. Until now, treating this dangerous disease was limited to supportive measures. But a new drug, ribavirin (Virazole), effectively treats the virus—not just its symptoms—by inhibiting protein synthesis.

Indicated for certain hospitalized infants and young children with severe lower respiratory tract infection from RSV, ribavirin is delivered directly to the lungs in aerosol mist form. A specially designed small-particle aerosol generator delivers the drug to the patient, who's under a hood or tent.

For best results, begin therapy within the first 3 days of RSV infection, and provide standard supportive measures to maintain respiratory function and fluid balance. For specific administration guidelines, see the chart below.

---

ribavirin (Virazole)

Mechanism of action
Inhibits viral activity by an unknown mechanism. Thought to inhibit RNA and DNA synthesis by depleting intracellular nucleotide pools.

Indication & dosage
Treatment of hospitalized infants and young children infected by RSV.
Infants and young children: Solution in concentration of 20 mg/ml delivered via the Viratek Small Particle Aerosol Generator (SPAG-2). Treatment is carried out for 12 to 18 hours/day for at least 3, and no more than 7, days.

Adverse reactions
• Blood: anemia, reticulocytosis
• Cardiovascular: cardiac arrest, hypotension
• Other: worsening of respiratory status, bacterial pneumonia, pneumothorax, apnea, ventilator dependence

Nursing considerations
• Ribavirin is contraindicated in women or girls who are or may become pregnant during exposure to the drug.
• Ribavirin is contraindicated in infants and children who need ventilatory assistance—ribavirin may precipitate in the respiratory equipment, inhibiting ventilation.
• Ribavirin aerosol is indicated only for lower respiratory tract infection caused by RSV. Although treatment may be started while awaiting diagnostic test results, RSV infection must be documented eventually.
• Most infants and children with RSV infection don't require treatment because the disease is often mild and self-limited. Those with such underlying conditions as prematurity or cardiopulmonary disease will benefit best from ribavirin therapy because they get the disease in its most severe form.
• Ribavirin aerosol *must* be administered by the Viratek SPAG-2. Don't use any other aerosol-generating device.
• The water used to solubilize the drug must not have any antimicrobial agent added. Use sterile USP water for injection, *not* bacteriostatic water.
• Discard solutions placed in the SPAG-2 unit at least every 24 hours before adding newly reconstituted solution.
• Store reconstituted solutions at room temperature for 24 hours.

Using the Babe-Shade Infant Ambient Light Reducer

If you're up on the latest research, you may know that premature infants exposed to ambient nursery light have a higher risk of retinopathy. To reduce this risk, Rocky Mountain Medical Corporation (RMMC) has developed the Babe-Shade Infant Ambient Light Reducer—soft, dark glasses that filter out two thirds of ambient light. With Babe-Shade, the infant can see, and nurses can keep nursery lights bright enough for infant monitoring.

Easy to apply and remove, the shade permits frequent eye contact, eye care, and examination. Because it doesn't use a constricting headband, it's safe even for an infant with a scalp I.V. And it's so soft that the infant can lie in any position. Important: Don't use Babe-Shade for an infant undergoing phototherapy for hyperbilirubinemia. Instead, use a standard opaque phototherapy mask, such as the RMMC Photo-Mask.

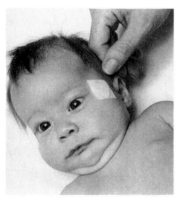

1 First, cleanse the infant's skin at his temples and around his eyes and ears. (To protect a premature infant's sensitive skin, you may also want to apply a skin barrier, such as Op-Site or HolliHesive Skin Barrier.) Then remove the Velcro heart strip from the package. Peel the paper from the tape square behind two of the hearts and gently press one square next to each eye.

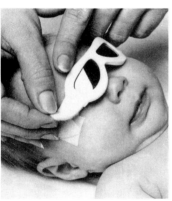

2 Apply Babe-Shade by pressing one of its ends to a heart and pulling the shade gently over the infant's eyes. Then press the other end to the second heart.

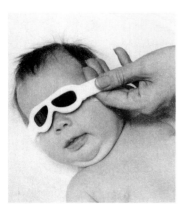

3 To examine the infant's eyes, hold one heart in place while lifting that end of the Shade, as the nurse is doing here. When the infant no longer needs Babe-Shade, remove it by loosening the hearts' tape backing with mineral or baby oil.

Treating growth hormone deficiency with somatrem

A biosynthetic growth hormone, somatrem (Protropin) offers new hope for children with growth hormone deficiency. Until 1985, such children routinely received human pituitary-derived growth hormone (pit-hGH) to help them achieve normal adult height. However, this therapy was discontinued by September 1985 after reports that at least three children being treated with pit-hGH had developed Jakob-Creutzfeldt disease, a rare, fatal viral infection causing spongiform cerebellar degeneration.

Created with recombinant DNA techniques, somatrem has performed well in clinical trials, tripling the average growth rate of children with growth hormone deficiency during the first year of therapy and more than doubling growth rates during the second and third years.

The sooner somatrem therapy begins, the more likely a child is to achieve normal adult height. The drug's effective only until linear bone growth stops and the epiphyses close—usually at the end of puberty.

For more details on somatrem therapy, see the following chart.

---

somatrem (Protropin)

Mechanism of action
Purified growth hormone of recombinant DNA origin that stimulates linear, skeletal, muscle, and organ growth.

Indication & dosage
Long-term treatment of children who lack adequate endogenous growth hormone secretion. *Children* (prepuberty): 0.1 mg/kg I.M. given three times weekly.

Adverse reactions
● Endocrine: hypothyroidism, hyperglycemia
● Other: antibodies to growth hormone

Interactions
Glucocorticoids may inhibit growth-promoting action of somatrem. Adjust the glucocorticoid dose, as ordered.

Nursing considerations
● Somatrem is contraindicated in patients with closed epiphyses, in patients who have an active underlying intracranial lesion, and in patients with a known sensitivity to benzyl alcohol.
● Use cautiously in patients whose growth hormone deficiency results from an intracranial lesion. The patient should be examined frequently for progression or recurrence of the underlying disease process.
● To prepare the solution, inject the bacteriostatic water for injection (which is supplied) into the vial containing the drug. Then swirl the vial with a gentle rotary motion until the contents completely dissolve. *Don't shake* the vial.
● After reconstitution, the vial solution should be clear. Don't inject it into the patient if the solution is cloudy or contains particles.
● Store the reconstituted drug in the refrigerator. Use it within 7 days.
● Be sure to check the expiration date before giving the drug.
● Observe the patient for signs of glucose intolerance and hyperglycemia.
● Monitor periodic thyroid function tests for hypothyroidism. If hypothyroidism occurs, the doctor will treat it with a thyroid hormone.
● Closely monitor a patient being treated for coexisting growth hormone deficiency and adrenocorticotropic hormone deficiency. A glucocorticoid prescribed to treat the latter condition may inhibit somatrem's growth-stimulating properties. The doctor must adjust glucocorticoid dosage precisely to ensure optimum growth.

Acknowledgments

We'd like to thank the clinical consultants from the following companies:

Abbott Laboratories
Hospital Products Division
Routes 137 & 43
Abbott Park, Ill. 60064

Ackrad Laboratories, Inc.
70 Jackson Drive
P.O. Box 1085
Cranford, N.J. 07016

American Edwards Laboratories
P.O. Box 11150
Santa Ana, Calif. 92711-1150

American Hospital Supply Corp.
6600 W. Touhy Avenue
Chicago, Ill. 60648

Ballard Medical Products
6864 S. 300 West
Midvale, Utah 84047

C.R. Bard, Inc.
Bard Cardiosurgery Division
P.O. Box M
Billerica, Mass. 01821

C.R. Bard, Inc.
Bard MedSystems Division
558 Central Avenue
Murray Hill, N.J. 07974

Becton Dickinson Vacutainer Systems
Stanely Street
Rutherford, N.J. 07070

Biosynergy, Inc.
724 W. Algonquin Road
Arlington Heights, Ill. 60005

Cardiac Pacemakers, Inc.
4100 N. Hamline Avenue
P.O. Box 64079
St. Paul, Minn. 55164

Cardiac Resuscitator Corp.
12244 S.W. Garden Place
Portland, Ore. 97223

Cormed, Inc.
591 Mahar Street
Medina, N.Y. 14103-1658

Dacomed Speech Systems
1701 E. 79th Street
Minneapolis, Minn. 55420

Danninger Medical Technology, Inc.
880 Kinnear Road
Columbus, Ohio 43212

Deknatel
Division of Pfizer Hospital Products Group, Inc.
110 Jericho Turnpike
Floral Park, N.Y. 11001

Genetic Laboratories, Inc.
1385 Centennial Drive
St. Paul, Minn. 55113

Healthdyne, Inc.
2253 Northwest Parkway
Marietta, Ga. 30067

Intelligent Medical Systems
Carlsbad Research Center
2233 Faraday Avenue
Suite K
Carlsbad, Calif. 92008-3849

Ivac Corp.
10300 Campus Point Drive
San Diego, Calif. 92121

The Kendall Company
Hospital Products
One Federal Street
Boston, Mass. 02101

Mammatech Corp.
930 N.W. 8th Avenue
Gainesville, Fla. 32601

Marion Laboratories, Inc.
Marion Scientific Division
P.O. Box 8480
Kansas City, Mo. 64114

Mediscus Products, Inc.
6700 E. Pacific Coast Highway
Suite 290
Long Beach, Calif. 90803

Medtronic, Inc.
7000 Central Avenue, N.E.
Minneapolis, Minn. 55432

Milex Products, Inc.
5915 N.W. Highway
Chicago, Ill. 60631

Minntech Corp.
Division of Renal Systems
14905 28th Avenue, N.
Minneapolis, Minn. 55441

Mon-a-therm, Inc.
500 S. Ewing Avenue
St. Louis, Mo. 63103

MorTan, Inc.
P.O. Drawer 1137
Torrington, Wyo. 82240

Nellcor, Inc.
25495 Whitesell Street
Hayward, Calif. 94545

Omni-Flow, Inc.
317 New Boston Street
Wilmington, Mass. 01887

Physio-Control Corp.
11811 Willows Road, N.E.
Redmond, Wash. 98073-9706

Puritan-Bennett Corp.
Bennett Division
2310 Camino Vida Roble
Carlsbad, Calif. 92008

Respironics, Inc.
530 Seco Road
Monroeville, Pa. 15146

Rocky Mountain Medical Corp.
5680 Greenwood Plaza Boulevard
Greenwood Village, Colo. 80111-2415

Roho, Inc.
P.O. Box 658
Belleville, Ill. 62222

Sarns, Inc./3M
6200 Jackson Road
Ann Arbor, Mich. 48103

Sherwood Medical, Inc.
Hospital Products Division
33 Benedict Place
Greenwich, Conn. 06830

Shiley Infusaid, Inc.
1400 Providence Highway
Norwood, Mass. 02062

SpectraScan, Inc.
45 S. Satellite Road
S. Windsor, Conn. 06074

Tokos Medical Corp.
1821 E. Dyer Road
Santa Ana, Calif. 92705

Trademark Corp.
1053 Headquarters Park
Fenton, Mo. 63026

Trilling Resources, Ltd.
250 E. Hartsdale Avenue
Hartsdale, N.Y. 10530

VLI Corp.
2031 Main Street
Irvine, Calif. 92714

Wyeth Laboratories, Inc.
P.O. Box 8299
Philadelphia, Pa. 19101

ZMI Corp.
325 Vassar Street
Cambridge, Mass. 02139

We'd also like to thank:

Community Ambulance Association
Station 351
P.O. Box 98
Ambler, Pa. 19002

Grandview Hospital
7000 Lawn Avenue
Sellersville, Pa. 18960
Barbara Bitros, RN

Hausted
927 Lake Road
Medina, Ohio 44258

McVan Pharmacy, Inc.
Lansdale, Pa. 19446
John McVan, Pharmacist

Simmons Health Care
P.O. Box 7247
Charlotte, N.C. 29217

WJS Healthcare
921 Thorne Drive
West Chester, Pa. 19382
Bill Burt

Selected References

American Heart Association. "Standards and Guidelines for Cardiopulmonary Resuscitation and Emergency Cardiac Care," *Journal of the American Medical Association* 255(21):2841-3044, June 6, 1986.

Beaver, Melissa J. "Mediscus Low Air-Loss Beds and the Prevention of Decubitus Ulcers," *Critical Care Nurse* 6(5):32-39, September/October 1986.

Brodsky, Jay B., et al. "Pulse Oximetry During One-Lung Ventilation," *Anesthesiology* 63(2):212-14, August 1985.

Cummins, R.O., et al. "What Is a 'Save'? Outcome Measures in Clinical Evaluations of Automatic External Defibrillators,"*American Heart Journal,* January, 1986.

Ersek, Robert A., et al. "New Natural Wound Dressing," *Physical Therapy Forum with Occupational Therapy Forum* 5(5):1-4, January 29, 1986.

Guarda, Nilda P., and Peterson, Janice Z. "If Your Patient Must Undergo Fine-Needle Biopsy," *RN* 49(10):34-35, October 1986.

Hughes, Carol B. "A Totally Implantable Central Venous System for Chemotherapy Administration: Nursing Considerations," *National Intravenous Therapy Association* 8(6):523-27, November/December 1985.

Hussar, Daniel A. "New Drugs," *Nursing86* 16(6):49-56, June 1986.

Katz, M., et al. "Assessment of Uterine Activity in Ambulatory Patients at High Risks of Preterm Labor and Delivery," *American Journal of Obstetrics and Gynecology* 154(1):44, January 1986.

Klug, Ruth Maring. "Children With AIDS," *American Journal of Nursing* 86(10):1126-32, October 1986.

Koop, C. Everett. "Surgeon General's Report on Acquired Immune Deficiency Syndrome," *Journal of the American Medical Association* 256(20):2784-89, November 28, 1986.

Kyba, Ferne Newman, et al. "Imaging: The Latest in Diagnostic Technology," *Nursing87* 17(1):45-47, January 1987.

Moorthy, S.S., et al. "Monitoring Urinary Bladder Temperature," *Heart & Lung* 14(1):90-93, January 1985.

Newhouse, Michael T., and Dolovich, Myrna B. "Control of Asthma by Aerosols," *New England Journal of Medicine* 315(14):870-73, October 2, 1986.

Noel, Debra K., et al. "Challenging Concerns for Patients with Automatic Implantable Cardioverter Defibrillators," *Focus on Critical Care* 13(6):50-57, December 1986.

Nursing87 Drug Handbook. Springhouse, Pa.: Springhouse Corp., 1987.

Nursing Yearbook87. Springhouse, Pa.: Springhouse Corp., 1987.

Palmer, Joyce Cotton, et al. "Nursing Management of Continuous Arteriovenous Hemofiltration for Acute Renal Failure," *Focus on Critical Care* 13(5):21-30, October 1986.

"A Place for Plasmapheresis," *Emergency Medicine* 18(21):73-86, December 15, 1986.

Quinn, Andrea. "Thora-Drain III: Closed Chest Drainage Made Simpler and Safer," *Nursing86* 16(9):46-51, September 1986.

Rahr, Virginia. "Giving Intrathecal Drugs...Ommaya Reservoirs," *American Journal of Nursing* 86(7):829-31, July 1986.

Ritz, Ray, et al. "Contamination of a Multiple-Use Suction Catheter in a Closed-Circuit System Compared to Contamination of a Disposable, Single-Use Suction Catheter," *Respiratory Care* 31(11):1086-91, November 1986.

Thurer, R.J., et al. "Automatic Implantable Cardioverter-Defibrillator: Techniques of Implantation and Results," *Annals of Thoracic Surgery* 42:143-47, 1986.

Wolff, Patricia Hooper, and Colletti, MaryAnn. "AIDS: Getting Past the Diagnosis and on to Discharge Planning," *Critical Care Nurse* 6(4):76-79, July/August 1986.

Young, Donald S. "Implementation of SI Units for Clinical Laboratory Data," *Annals of Internal Medicine* 106(1):114-29, January 1987.

Zoll, Paul M., et al. "External Noninvasive Temporary Cardiac Pacing: Clinical Trials," *Circulation* 71(5):937-44, May 1985.

Index

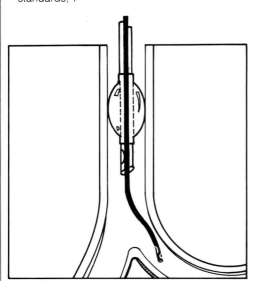

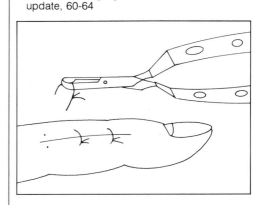

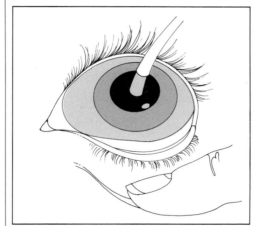

Index

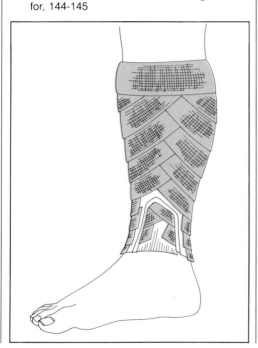